ALTERNATIVE
CAREERS
IN SCIENCE

• • • • • • • • • •

Leaving the Ivory Tower

Second Edition

ALTERNATIVE CAREERS IN SCIENCE

Leaving the Ivory Tower

Second Edition

Edited by

Cynthia Robbins-Roth

ELSEVIER
ACADEMIC
PRESS

AMSTERDAM • BOSTON • HEIDELBERG • LONDON
NEW YORK • OXFORD • PARIS • SAN DIEGO
SAN FRANCISCO • SINGAPORE • SYDNEY • TOKYO

Elsevier Academic Press

30 Corporate Drive, Suite 400, Burlington, MA 01803, USA
525 B Street, Suite 1900, San Diego, California 92101-4495, USA
84 Theobald's Road, London WC1X 8RR, UK

This book is printed on acid-free paper. ⊚

Library of Congress Cataloging-in-Publication Data
Application submitted.

British Library Cataloguing in Publication Data
A catalogue record for this book is available from the British Library

ISBN 13: 978-0-12-589376-3
ISBN 10: 0-12-589376-0

For all information on all Elsevier Academic Press publications
visit our Web site at www.books.elsevier.com

Printed in the United States of America
05 06 07 08 09 10 11 9 8 7 6 5 4 3 2 1

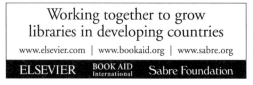

Working together to grow
libraries in developing countries

www.elsevier.com | www.bookaid.org | www.sabre.org

ELSEVIER   BOOK AID   Sabre Foundation
            International

TABLE OF CONTENTS

· · · · · · · · · · · · · · · · · ·

PROVIDING SERVICES TO COMPANIES
•••••••••••••••••••••••••

CONTRIBUTORS

Numbers in parenthesis indicate the pages on which the author's contributions begin.

DAVID APPELGATE (245), U.S. Geological Survey, Reston, Virginia 20192

ALEXANDRA J. BARAN (139), A.J. Baran Consulting Inc., Palo Alto, California 94025

RON COHEN (97), Acorda Therapeutics, New York, New York 10532

MARK D. DIBNER (47), BioAbility, Research Triangle Park, North Carolina 27709

PETER DRAKE (71), Mayflower Partners, Chicago, Illinois 60610

SUE GOETINCK AMBROSE (27), The Dallas Morning News, Dallas, Texas 75214

MARY ANN GRAY (79), Gray Strategic Advisors, New York, New York 10023

GENEVIEVE HADDAD (277), Air Force Office of Scientific Research, Bolling Air Force Base, Washington, D.C. 20332

CAROL HALL (217), BioVenture Consultants, Chestnut Hill, Massachusetts 02467

PHILIP W. HAMMER (117), The Franklin Center, The Franklin Institute Science Museum, Philadelphia, Pennsylvania 19103

BENTE HANSEN (205), Bente Hansen & Associates, San Diego, California 92130

GINA LENTO (263), New Zealand Trade & Enterprise, Auckland, New Zealand

ROGER LONGMAN (39), Windover Information, Inc., South Norwalk, Connecticut 06856

ERIN HALL MEADE (161), Life Alaska Donor Services, Anchorage, Alaska 99507

ELIZABETH D. MOYER (125), M/P Biomedical Consultants, LLC, Mill Valley, California 94941

DEEPA PAKIANATHAN (61), Delphi Bioventures, Menlo Park, California 94025

RONALD PEPIN (107), Medarex, Inc., Princeton, New Jersey 08543

CLAYTON R. RANDALL (15), Formerly with PE Applied Systems, Foster City, California 94404

CYNTHIA ROBBINS-ROTH (1, 291), BioVenture Consultants, San Mateo, California 94403

ROBERT ROTH (149), THE WEINBERG GROUP INC., San Francisco, California 94105

TONY RUSSO (191), Noonan Russo, Euro RSCG NRP, New York, New York 10016

GAIL SCHECHTER (227), BioIntelligence, San Francisco, California 94115

PAULA SZOKA (177), University of Washington Technology Transfer, University of Washington, Seattle, Washington 98105

PREFACE

When I began my path toward becoming an academic scientist back in college, I never dreamed that I would stray so far from that expected fate. My travels took me through worlds I had never even considered—business development, journalism, publishing, running small businesses, and being an independent consultant. While I wandered far from my original objective, science remained the core motivation behind all of these career changes. Even today, several decades after I began my biology major at Bates College (Lewiston, Maine), my love of discovery, learning about new areas of science, and spending time with scientists is the core driver for all of my activities. The only real change is that my focus is now bringing that science into the rest of the world.

When I began this voyage there were few road signs to follow—biological scientists simply did not leave the academic lab back in the 1970s and early 1980s. I had to forge my own path from the bench to the boardroom. Today, I have the chance to be a mentor to others who are making the same trip. My fellow "scientists gone bad" and I are deluged with phone calls and e-mails from graduate students, post-doctorates, tenured professors, and industry scientists who, for a wide range of reasons, are looking for clues to life outside the lab. I hope this book inspires them to make the leap.

This book is dedicated to all of those who helped me in my evolution, and most especially to Dr. Steve Bennett, the M.D./Ph.D. who first led me into the world of venture capital; Brook Byers, who helped build an entire new industry around science and who supported my early writing activities; Dr. Stelios Papadopoulos, and academic scientist turned banker who helped finance that new industry; Joan O'C. Hamilton, who taught me important lessons about journalism; Dr. Steve Spencer, who watched way too many episodes of *The A Team* with me as I tortured myself over leaving the lab; Stefan Borg, who bravely turned a bench scientist into a business development maven; Dr. Carol Hall, my longtime friend and partner in BioVenture Consultants, who forced me to see the beauty in finance and the synergy achieved by two diverse minds working together; and most of all, my husband, Robert Roth, an M.D./Ph.D. whose love and support gave me courage as I headed into uncharted territory—and who has since made that same journey himself.

Chapter

1

••••••••••

A SCIENTIST GONE BAD:

How I Went from the Bench to the Board Room

•••••••••••••••••

Cynthia Robbins-Roth, Ph.D.
Principal, BioVenture Consultants

It all began so innocently—back in 1984, I was happily running gels and killing tumors in mice. One year later, I was wearing grown-up clothes and hanging out with vice presidents and chief executive officers.

After that first move out of the lab, I founded *BioVenture View*, a monthly biotech industry newsletter, and *BioPeople Magazine*, the first biotech industry magazine about the movers and shakers building the sector; I became founding editor of *BioWorld Today*, the first daily online/faxed biotech newsletter; I started BioVenture Consultants, which still provides business, technology, and financial consulting services to start-up businesses and established biopharmaceutical ("biopharma") companies around the globe; I started writing a regular biotech industry column for *Forbes Magazine* and *Forbes ASAP*, along with two books (this book and *From Alchemy to IPO: The Business of Biotechnology*). You probably noticed that *bio* is part of all of these endeavors. That early scientific bent remained a big part of all that I do. I have traveled throughout North America, Europe, and the Pacific Rim, giving invited talks and working with governments and young companies. And yet, I haven't done a hands-on experiment since 1984.

And I couldn't be happier.

This completely unplanned-for transition has led me into a universe of opportunities to earn my living by spending time with world-class researchers pushing back the frontier of science and by communicating the excitement and promise of that technology to the rest of the world. And what other biochemist can claim to have been quoted in that respected scientific journal *Town & Country*?

When I crossed that line from scientist to "suit," there were very few examples for me to study. Researchers in the biological sciences were just starting to believe that it might be okay to leave academia and go into the newly emerging biotech industry—but only as a scientist! I had no idea what a scientist could do outside of the lab. I had spent my entire career immersed in a very rarefied environment, surrounded by other biomedical researchers who saw the simple move from university to company lab as the most radical career move ever!

These days, with government funding for academic research still very much under pressure, with a dearth of academic jobs (with or without tenure!), and with a growing sense that there must be more possibilities out there, graduate students and other members of the academic community are beginning their search for life after lab much earlier. I find that many universities have active career seminar series that bring students and faculty into contact with former scientists who have entered a diverse range of careers. Many corporate scientists are looking for ways to grow beyond the lab.

This book gives you the insider's story on 24 different ways to put that scientific training to good use away from the lab bench and away from academia. Each of our authors took an unexpected detour into worlds that were previously unimagined during their early training. And while each of these jobs took the authors far from their original paths, the key to their success and enjoyment of new careers was the critical role science continued to play.

Right now, it might be tough to see how a scientific background could be valuable to a stock analyst, publisher, or government policy expert. But, as you will learn from these personal stories, it's the science that taught them all to think analytically, to structure an approach to new areas, and to forge ahead into new territory without fear (or at least not much fear).

The world is full of those with M.B.A.s who long to enter the growing biotech sector but who just can't master the intricacies of the technology sufficiently to be useful to the companies or investors; of patent lawyers who struggle with applications because they can't fully grasp the prior art in the scientific literature; and of information providers who don't understand the information they sell and thus can't always tell the difference between crucial and just interesting data.

Don't let anyone tell you that science is a dead end, now that becoming a full-tenured professor seems out of reach. And don't believe anyone who tells you that it is a waste of time to pursue a science education unless you plan to stay in the lab. There is a wide universe out there, just waiting for you to explore!

"And do not believe anyone who tells you that it is a waste of time to pursue a science education unless you plan to stay in the lab."

SO HOW DID THIS HAPPEN?

I was first bitten by the science bug in seventh grade. The teacher was showing us how dripping acid on a rock could determine if it was lime-stone. This simple-minded experiment had a huge impact on me. I loved the idea that you could do experiments to figure out something that you didn't already know, that you could query the universe! This appealed to me immensely, in part because I already had a serious problem with authority figures and loved the idea that you could find answers independently.

While the specific field of interest evolved for me over time, the basic drive toward lab work never changed. At Bates College, my biochemistry focus shifted a bit when I took my first immunology course, taught by a young scientist fresh out of his post-doctoral position ("post-doc") at Yale. Immunology was just on the verge of converting from phenomenology (okay, stick this stuff into a bunny and see what happens!) into a realm where a protein biochemist could have some fun and learn cool new stuff about how the immune system actually worked. That teacher was the first to let me into the wonderful world of hands-on science—I was in love.

I moved to the University of Texas Medical Branch in Galveston for my Ph.D. work with Dr. Benjamin Papermaster, whose lab was focused on applying the tools of biochemistry to purify and characterize the proteins that carry messages (Kill that tumor! Wipe out the virally infected cell!) for the immune system. I was intrigued with the idea that we could use our work to find a way to provide cancer patients with the immune factors their own systems were not making, moving away from the incredibly toxic chemotherapy drugs that were the only treatment available at the time.

By 1980, it became increasingly clear that, while I loved the lab work, academia was not for me. If I had to listen to one more medical student whine about the lab work I had to teach them, I would be forced to throw them through a window—which would probably be detrimental to my academic career. I started interviewing for jobs at pharmaceutical companies, but I was discouraged by their overpopulation of middle-aged white guys in clean lab coats and ties who all went home at 4:30 in the afternoon. These companies seemed too conservative for me, and my little problem with authority figures had not gone away.

In 1980, while I was in the midst of a post-doc in the interferon lab of Dr. Howard Johnson, I got a phone call from a scientist at a newly formed company—Genentech, Inc., in southern San Francisco, California. While I had no idea what this "biotech" industry was, my ears perked up when he said the company was only 2 years old and had chosen cytokines—my area of interest—as an initial research focus. We agreed to meet in Paris at the week-long International Immunology Congress (really, ALL job interviews should take place in Paris, don't you think?). To this day, I am convinced it was my ability to order him his first full meal in French that got me the job.

In spite of howls of "traitor" from my academic colleagues, Genentech turned out to be exactly what I was looking for, in many ways. The labs were packed with young ex-post-docs and those with recently received Ph.D. titles who had no commercial experience, along with just about every piece of equipment you could want. The company environment was very entrepreneurial—Genentech was one of the first biotech companies formed, and it changed the ground rules for doing science in a corporate setting. Dress codes were nonexistent, scientists kept whatever schedules they wanted (being ex-post-docs, we all worked 18-hour days, at least 6 days a week), and we didn't have to write grants or teach medical students! I was working with some of the best scientists in a broad range of disciplines—protein chemistry, immunology, tumor biology, molecular biology, X-ray crystallography, assay development, and so on. I was in heaven.

At Genentech, my "jack-of-all-trades, master of none" personality, first nurtured in Johnson's lab, really came into play. While I was supposed to be focused exclusively on assay design and purification schemes, I spent a lot of time wandering the halls and learning how to do amino acid composition and sequencing, RNA purification (and why you really don't want phenol on your hands), and some really hard-core protein biochemistry. I learned about the problems in designing productive animal studies and the challenges a young entrepreneurial company faced when starting with 75 folks, who knew each other pretty well, and ending up with 150 people and more.

During my Genentech stint, I spent time as a project team leader. The phrase "herding cats" springs to mind when remembering what it was like to get a group of aggressive, competitive scientists from different departments to quit bickering and start cooperating so that the project could move forward. This experience convinced me that people management skills—not just excellent science—were crucial to a successful business and that I needed to improve my people skills!

HEADING OUT OF THE LAB

That other change in my thought process was the realization that science for its own sake wasn't all that satisfying for me. I wanted my work to contribute to developing a new therapeutic treatment that could help patients. I wanted to understand how the company decided which science projects would generate the best products and what issues outside of technical points had to be considered.

As luck would have it, my incredible ineptness at corporate politics and frustration with the "pushing limp spaghetti" aspect of team building in a nonteam environment propelled me out of the lab and into the best place to learn the answers to my questions—business development.

I wanted desperately to leave Genentech and the constant battles, but I couldn't find a bench job that wasn't in conflict with my project at Genentech. I had no idea how to find a nonbench job. The only scientist I knew who had made the transition was another biochemist with a Ph.D. who became a patent lawyer—but the idea of going to law school did not appeal to me at all.

I started scanning the newspaper want ads and reading the classified ads in the back of *Science* and *Nature*. Months went by before I stumbled on an ad for "Advisor to the CEO" at a company I had never heard of, California Biotechnology, Inc., in Mountain View. I had no idea what they did there, but what the heck, they were looking for a scientist with a Ph.D., someone with biotech experience, and I certainly could give advice! (Of course, I worried that my shy and retiring personality might be a drawback.)

I sent a résumé and was invited for an interview. It turned out the Cal Bio was a biotherapeutic company with 75 employees and 35 ongoing projects. The CEO wanted me to help analyze the huge number of projects and help the management team determine which were great product opportunities and which were not—my first exposure to the concept of due diligence.

The perfect job! I had to learn how to analyze science not just from the perspective of experimental design and data but also through examining intellectual property issues and competition from other biotech firms and "big pharma" companies (large, sometimes multinational, pharmaceutical companies). I had to build a network of clinicians to learn what they saw as critical medical problems requiring a novel approach; I had to understand what it would take to develop such a product from lab to FDA approval and into the marketplace.

Luckily, I had a great mentor, Stefan Borg. He had a molecular biology background plus an M.B.A. degree. Stefan taught me the basics of business development and encouraged me on a daily basis.

I loved it! My science training in tracking down information and fitting pieces of data together to form a picture came in very handy, along with the ability to critically evaluate and analytically work through a problem to obtain a potentially unexpected answer. Because the 35 projects were in such a wide range of clinical settings, I had to conquer a broad range of disciplines. It was my job to track down experts in various fields and entice them into telling me everything I needed to know. In other words, I got paid to be educated in many new areas by the experts—what a great deal!

"I got paid to be educated in many new areas by the experts—what a great deal!"

I found that my scientific background and degree were almost more important than any growing business sense. Just mentioning these things gave me instant credibility with wary scientists who were getting really tired of talking to nonscientists—the bankers, analysts, lawyers, and corporate executives who wanted to put their inventions to work.

COMMUNICATION SKILLS BECOME IMPORTANT

As I started putting together my reports to the management team on these projects, I found that I had to communicate the key concepts and issues in a language that they understood. If the CEO did not grasp the gist of my recommendations, all that work was useless to the company, no matter how profound my analysis. This basic fact of life forced me to improve my writing skills, which consisted solely of knowing how to write dry journal articles for other scientists in my very narrow field. In the process, I found that I loved to write, and I loved finding ways to communicate to others my excitement about an area of science.

This led me in 1984 to start an in-house newsletter—*The RR Report*—to keep management informed about the activities of competing biotech and pharmaceutical firms and to highlight interesting scientific papers and conference presentations that might be interesting for the company. I had to learn how to use word processing programs to generate my reports and the newsletter—the departmental secretary informed me that she "didn't work for girls." I learned how to build database programs because it was the only way to keep track of the information in my newsletters. Although I whined about having to learn this stuff back then, it gave me the confidence to tackle computer hardware and software (it also taught me to avoid reading manuals).

This little newsletter brought me to the attention of Dr. Steve Bennett, a physician and scientist from Stanford and the World Health Organization who had been recruited to run the medical portfolio of G.T. Capital's Emerging Technologies fund. Steve was an important investor in Cal Bio and felt it was a great idea to put a scientist with a Ph.D. in business development (a weird idea then, fairly common now). He introduced himself, and that was the beginning of a beautiful friendship. He also introduced me to Dr. Carol Hall, a scientist turned Wall Street analyst, who got me thinking about the role of public investors in biotech.

ONCE MORE INTO THE FRAY—GOING INDEPENDENT

In 1986, when I found myself on the wrong side of company politics yet again and decided that perhaps I just wasn't cut out to be an employee, I met with Steve to discuss my future. I had a job offer—a significant promotion over my Cal Bio position—but I was resisting. Steve's answer was, "So become a consultant! In fact, come work for my fund." And so I took another great leap into self-employment and the wild world of venture capital. The strong support of my husband, still ensconced in the academic science world, gave me the guts to try.

Once again, an unplanned move turned out to be the perfect place for me. The flexibility of working for myself was a blessing because I had a 6-month-old son. I loved working with Steve's fund, which was heavily invested in both public and private biotech firms. Steve taught me to understand some of the issues and agendas that investors must face, especially fund managers and venture capitalists who have their own investors and limited partners who whine about return on investment. He also showed me just what a great investor can bring to a company besides money. He was an active participant on boards of directors of several of his portfolio companies and actively stayed in touch with others.

The 1980s were heady days for biotech venture investing. Through Steve and at his office at 3000 Sand Hill Road, I met and worked with many of the key players. I admired the way this first generation of biotech venture capitalists focused on building successful operating businesses around this emerging new technology. The rocky ride on Wall Street made financing a challenge, and the long product development time frame made smart management critical for survival. The venture capitalists (VCs) taught me how to pay attention to a broad range of key issues and not just remain enamored with the sexy science.

I thrived on the chaos and uncertainty of independent consulting. I loved working on multiple projects simultaneously. I had the chance to interact with a huge number of very smart people and developed a powerful network of folks in and around the industry. I learned quickly that you always try to treat people fairly and help out when you can—you never know when and where that person will show up again! The phrase "what goes around, comes around" is really true.

PUBLISHING GETS ADDED TO THE MIX

But even as I became immersed in the consulting world, I was starting a second business—an industry newsletter. After I had worked with Steve's firm for about a month, he suggested that the *RR Report*, my Cal Bio in-house newsletter, would make a great publication for the venture community investing in this emerging industry. He offered me free run of the G.T. Capital office to work on the newsletter, including access to computers, printers, copiers, and the all-important postage machine. And so *BioVenture View* (*BVV*), the first newsletter to focus on the business of biotechnology, was launched in mid-1986 in the hotbed of biotech venture capital on Sand Hill Road.

The consulting and publishing sides of my business were a great synergistic fit—my monthly writing fits improved my writing skills considerably, and the increasing flow of company news into my files gave me a growing database of information for the consulting business. The key was keeping an absolutely strict confidentiality in place—no consulting client ever found their confidential information on the pages of *BioVenture View*.

As the newsletter grew in circulation, spreading to executives in the venture-backed firms and then to the wider biotech community, I was struggling to keep up with the business. I spent my evenings and weekends on the living room floor, stuffing and sealing envelopes full of newsletters or renewal invoices. Carol Hall re-entered my life as a great commentator on the world of biotech finance and occasional *BVV* writer on financial topics. It was great to have someone else whose view of science and business was so complementary to mine. By late 1998, she quit her job at a leveraged buyout firm and joined me in BioVenture Consultants.

When my second child was about 6 months old, another change came. I was recruited by David Bunnell, a well-known publisher in the computer world, to help create *BioWorld*, the first daily online news and information service focused on the biotech industry. This change made me an employee again, although at least this time I was in charge of my domain— the editorial group—and was part of the "Gang of Four" that managed the company.

Running a daily newsroom was a complete change for me. I had to create a newsroom that could provide very specialized reporting. The pace was outrageous compared to the monthly crawl of *BioVenture View* (which I was still writing), and I had never worked before with professional journalists and copyeditors. We built a great news service that transformed coverage of the biotech world and made our industry suddenly very visible to the general public. We also created *BioWorld Magazine*, which gave me my first taste of the thrill of seeing great editorial teamed up with fantastic graphics.

While daily news can be very addictive, I started getting worn out from the relentless pace and chaffing associated with being an employee once again. In early 1991, I left *BioWorld* and took *BioVenture View* independent once again. A steady trickle of folks from *BioWorld* started showing up at World Headquarters, my office in the backyard. Together, we rebuilt *BioVenture View* and created *BioPeople Magazine*.

At the same time, Carol Hall and I revved BioVenture Consultants back up. Our client base evolved away from the venture capitalists and toward working directly with early-stage biotech firms on an international basis. We wrote business plans, helped with restarts of companies whose initial strategies didn't work out, assisted with public and private financings, helped find corporate partners, and generally had a great time.

As the consulting business grew, the networks that Carol and I had nurtured all those years paid off. They brought us great projects and access to experts whose input we and our clients needed. In many ways, we act as biotech yentas, matchmakers who look at science, financial issues, and management teams to bring together the critical mass for successful growth. We work with brand new firms; established multinational pharmaceutical companies; and groups in Canada, Asia, Australia, New Zealand, and Europe, as well as in the United States. Carol also became the editor of *BioVenture Stock Report*.

● ●
"I am invited all over the world to speak about aspects of the biotech industry and on alternative careers for scientists."
● ●

In 1996, I realized that my publishing business and BioVenture Consultants had both grown rapidly. I had to either grow my employee base past the five in-house staff members supporting our three publications or choose between the publishing and consulting sides of my business. I sold the publishing business to PJB Publications, a UK-based pharmaceutical publishing business, and focused on consulting.

I became even more involved with various industry companies, accepting two board of director seats with biotech start-ups and serving on the advisory boards for a Singapore venture fund and a Toronto-based seed venture fund. I am invited all over the world to speak about aspects of the biotech industry and on alternative careers for scientists. I still have the writing bug, which has led to regular writing gigs with *Forbes Magazine* and *Forbes ASAP*, with an Internet-based biotech investment newsletter, and the chance to write two books—this one that you are reading and one on the history and evolution of the biotech industry.

ALTERNATIVE CAREERS

Carol and I are both the beneficiaries of mentors who helped us find our way in new fields, and we field calls and e-mails every week from students, faculty, and industry folks investigating the possibilities outside the lab—or even outside other careers. More and more scientists are forced to consider alternatives to the classic academic track, thanks to the low supply of jobs. And people in many careers outside of the biotech world are lured by the excitement and promise of this new industry.

Even though I don't run gels and columns any more (and I am pretty sure I can't still perform cardiac puncture successfully), I very strongly believe that the key to my contribution to our clients and readers lies in my hard-core, hands-on science training. While I have spent the past 20 years learning many other disciplines, it is that core experience that informs how I think and analyze, how I bring together apparently disparate pieces of information. The driving force behind my enthusiasm for my work is my love of the science that lies behind it all.

This book is full of personal stories from individuals who share a strong scientific background. While they ended up in an amazingly diverse collection of jobs, there are certain recurring themes that you will find in all of their stories. The first is a willingness to take a chance, to give serendipity an opportunity to work. The second is a strong streak of self-confidence, the willingness to risk falling flat on their faces.

This doesn't mean that everything went smoothly for our authors. On the contrary, you will find that most of them faced real adversity. This very impediment to their expected path is what flung them into unexpected areas that they have come to love. All of these authors have learned how to build strong interpersonal relationships, even those of us who have problems taking orders! The ability to create a team—of mentors or staff with various backgrounds—allows you to make almost any transition.

I encourage all of you to pursue these far-flung opportunities and find some of your own. Oh, and remember that nice young post-doc who first set me loose in an unsuspecting laboratory? He is now wearing a suit himself, having moved from the lab into the Office of Science and Technology at Duke University, and currently he is vice president of technology at a biotech start-up that he helped build. His broad scientific knowledge and ability to understand the issues affecting all sides of negotiations between scientists, clinicians, the biopharmaceutical industry, and the financial community were important keys to his success.

So take off your lab coat, and check out this new universe. You never know where you might end up!

SCIENCE AND INFORMATION

Chapter

TECHNICAL WRITING:

Making Sense Out of Manuals

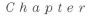

Clayton R. Randall, Ph.D.[*]

Former Senior Technical Writer, PE Applied Biosystems

WHAT IS A TECHNICAL WRITER?

The broadest definition of a technical writer is someone who compiles large quantities of information into a useful, easily digested form for a specific audience. A journalist for *Scientific American* is a technical writer; the person who writes instruction manuals for *Mathematica* or *Doom II* is a technical writer. So are you, if you have written scientific papers (although the "easily digested" part doesn't apply as much).

In the San Francisco Bay area where I live, most technical writers write manuals and online help files documenting computer software and hardware, although more jobs are becoming available in other fields such as biotechnology.

I work for the life science division of a large analytical instrument company that is the world's leading provider of DNA synthesis and analysis equipment and the reagent kits that are used on the equipment. I write instruction manuals for the reagent kits, which have specific applications, such as DNA sequencing, human identification from forensic evidence, and food testing for *Salmonella*.

[*]Updated for second edition by Cynthia Robbins-Roth

WHY TECH WRITING IS A GREAT MOVE

Here are some reasons why technical writing is a good career transition for scientists:

- You don't have to stop being a scientist. You still have daily contact with scientists and discuss their work with them. Besides, it is impossible to stop being a scientist. It is in the blood, and it is how we were trained to think. I often refer to myself as a "recovering scientist" because I left research but will always be a scientist.

- You have instant credibility with "subject matter experts." Because you are also a scientist, the scientists and engineers with whom you work think automatically that you know what you are doing. They don't think that way about all tech writers, which is a downside of the field. It is up to you to maintain that credibility by the way in which you perform your job.

- You don't have to do lab work. The endless repetition of experiments is one reason many of us left research. As a writer, you get to learn about new scientific methods and new software without having to do the grunt work of repetition and method validation. The thrill of learning is why I became a scientist—not because of the drudgery that can go along with it. When a tech writing project is done, you go on to the next project. You don't have to keep doing the same thing for years on end.

- You can still do some lab work if you want. The best way to learn about a new product is to test it, whether it is a reagent kit or piece of software. In fact, the product team will respect you greatly if you take the product for a test drive.

- You resemble the customers. As a biotechnology writer, I have a lot in common with the end users of my company's products, who are research scientists and technicians. One of my coworkers, another chemist who has a Ph.D., got her first job because she used certain computational software extensively. The software company needed a new manual at the same time her post-doc funding was running out. Because you resemble the customers, you understand their concerns and can write about what they want to know.

- You will have a learning curve that is less steep than will most writers. You already know a lot of science, and you have the background to learn more science easily. And don't forget that you are more computer literate than 95% of the population. Scientists use computers to collect their data, analyze it, and write up the results.

- Your work ethic will be appreciated. Most scientists work hard, are inquisitive, and pay close attention to detail. These are all useful qualities in technical writers. We need to go out and learn as much as possible about our subject and then make sure that we write carefully and accurately.

Overall, scientists and technical writing are a good fit. Your technical background, willingness to learn, and meticulousness will serve you well as a tech writer.

COMMON PERSONALITY TRAITS OF TECH WRITERS

Lifelong learning is the most important trait of a technical writer. You should be interested in almost everything and willing to learn as much as you can about it. If you are excited about your subject, your writing will be interesting as well.

You have to like writing. I realized that one of the things I consistently enjoyed about science was seeing my work in print. I also enjoyed explaining my work to my nonscientist friends, who always said that I was good at making science understandable. I discovered that there were people, called technical writers, who did this for a living. The idea of being paid good money to write was appealing.

"The idea of being paid good money to write was appealing."

You must enjoy working with people. Most of the information you use to write documentation comes from interviewing subject matter experts singly or in groups. Even if you are given a written draft of a procedure, you will still have to talk with its author to clarify and complete it. The networks you establish by trading information and favors are very important in getting your job done (more on networking later). It isn't necessary to be a complete extrovert, but you have to be able to talk to many different kinds of people. Take an interest in them and learn about them as well. It is part of what makes the job fun.

Pursue knowledge actively and be tenacious. You have to go out and find what you need rather than waiting for it to be dropped over your cubicle wall. If you don't get what you need the first time, go back and bother the necessary people again and again until they give you what you want just to get rid of you. They have their priorities, but so do you.

Pay close attention to detail, but don't be consumed by it. Your grammar and spelling must be flawless, and your content as accurate as possible, but don't try to write a perfect document. That takes too much time, and the product has to get out the door to make money so that everyone gets paid.

The ability to handle multiple tasks and projects simultaneously is crucial. It is common to work on several projects at once, each with its own issues and deadlines. Even if you work on only one or two large projects at once, each can have many chapters and bits of information to juggle.

Finally, it is actually good to have a short attention span. I am interested in almost everything, learn quickly, and get bored quickly. In grad school, I had trouble staying focused on the same project for years. Now, I work on several projects at once and finish 10 or 15 projects per year, ranging from 30-page reagent kit protocols to 250-page user's manuals. Mostly, I write shorter documents. When something is done, I move on.

On the other hand, some tech writers prefer working on larger projects for a longer period of time. They like to work on the same lengthy project for 6 months, a year, or longer. What would be anathema to me works for them. Still other tech writers fall somewhere between the two extremes and work on a variety of projects.

A Typical Day at Work

I usually get in between 9:00 and 9:30 A.M. I turn on my computer and, while it is booting up, check my voice mail to see what crises have arisen since I left the night before. If I have no voice mail, I get a cup of coffee, the first of two or three during the day. Once the computer's up, I check my e-mail and then spend some time talking with my coworkers, especially if it is Monday, and they have good stories from the weekend.

After returning phone calls and putting out fires, I spend most of the morning writing and editing, unless I need to get a manual to the printer or I have a meeting.

Writers in my department are responsible for all aspects of their documents, from planning to writing to getting the electronic deliverables (printable files) ready to send to the print vendor. I have also put some of my manuals on the company Web site. Each project team usually meets weekly to discuss progress, which means I have four to seven meetings each week, not including impromptu meetings called to review drafts of manuals or to handle sudden research or manufacturing issues. Projects, such as those concerning a new instrument or reagent kit, are accomplished by interdisciplinary teams composed of people from marketing, research, and development; process development; manufacturing; technical communications; and other such departments. There are also staff meetings, during which a department such as technical communications gets together to discuss the work week and what its people did since the last meeting.

After the morning writing and/or meetings, there is a lunch break. I usually go off-site with a few coworkers or one or two friends from other departments (we have a cafeteria, but I don't like the food). I met most of my friends in other departments by working on team projects with them. If I have just finished a project, I reward myself by going out for sushi. Celebrating accomplishments is important in any job.

After lunch, I check voice mail and e-mail again. (On a slow day, I check e-mail about 10 times.) The afternoon is spent like the morning: writing, editing, or going to meetings. I take some time to walk around and check with people in the various project teams if I need information from them or if I have information to share with them. I also return voice mail from people looking for a manual or for information that I have or that I might know where to find.

I enjoy networking, and I find that if I go out of my way to help other people, they will do the same for me. Because I work on many projects across the company, I know more of what is going on than do most people who work in only one department. I know about new projects before they are dropped on my desk.

• •
"I enjoy networking, and I find that if I go out of my way to help other people, they will do the same for me."
• •

After 5:00 P.M., our department gets quieter as people go home. I work for another hour or so, check the e-mail one last time, then leave around 6:00 or 6:30 P.M. We don't have set hours; we just have to get the work done.

What I Like Best About My Job

The best thing about my job is that I write creatively while helping people. They follow my instructions to use our company's reagent kits to test food for harmful bacteria, to find new genes, or to show which suspect could or could not have committed a crime. My work has very tangible results.

When I explain my job to my friends and relatives who aren't scientists, I tell them about the real-world applications of my work, adding that I "explain science to normal people." They immediately understand and approve. Try explaining the K_β X-ray fluorescence spectroscopy of metalloproteins (my post-doc work) and its utility (if any) to your relatives in less than 100 words. It doesn't work.

Technical writers help people do what they need to do. The corollary to this is that our work is read by many people. A friend of mine pointed out that my work is read and used by thousands or tens of thousands of scientists, more than any but the hottest papers in *Science* or *Nature*. Besides, I get to see my work in print 10 to 15 times a year.

On a more mundane level, I like being told that I have done a good job. That seems to happen more in industry than in academia, where instead you are told, "good work, but you need to repeat it and do five more studies like it."

What I Don't Like About My Job

Like any field, technical writing has its disadvantages. Some of them are common to other fields as well.

Repetitive stress injury (RSI) is the biggest job-related hazard for technical writers. Because we type and use the mouse (the most antiergonomic thing in existence other than high-heeled shoes and neckties) most of the day, our wrists and hands are particularly vulnerable. Eye strain and lower back strain can also occur. When working, take frequent breaks—at least once every half hour—especially if you are working a lot with a mouse. If your hand is often sore, you probably already have an RSI. If you have chronic pain, see your doctor.

Tech writers are also susceptible to stress, mainly because of deadlines and juggling too many projects at once. Frustration commonly occurs with project teams who think that your document is a much lower priority than you do and act accordingly. Frustration with project teams who think you are a glorified typist also occurs, although this attitude occurs less often for scientifically trained writers. Sometimes you also get frustrated with your boss, who wants the document to be perfect when you just want to get it out the door.

• • • • • • • • • • • • • • • • • • • •

"Tech writers are also susceptible to stress, mainly because of deadlines and juggling too many projects at once."

• •

Another source of frustration comes from paperwork. More and more companies are obtaining ISO 9000 certification, which states that the company follows certain written procedures consistently. ISO 9000 works well for manufacturing processes but not as well for technical documentation, where it can complicate your job unnecessarily. The problem often is not the standards themselves but how they are written. The people who write the standards seem to feel that because there must be standards, the standards must be complex. In this case, procedures can get in the way of doing your job.

COMPARISONS WITH THE ACADEMIC WORLD

How Is This Work Like Grad School And Post-Doc Work?

- **Skills:** Technical writing uses many of the same skills—analytical, scientific, and computer skills.

- **Challenges:** Writers are constantly learning new scientific procedures and how to master computer software.

- **Networking:** Writers have to make contacts to find out the information they need to do their work, to find out the latest advances in their company's field or in writing, and to find out where the good jobs are. This includes attending scientific or technical writing conferences.

How Is This Work Different from Grad School and Post-Doc Work?

- **Salary:** According to the Society for Technical Communication (sort of like the AAAS for tech writers), the average technical writer in the United States makes from $45,000 to $50,000 per year. In the Bay Area, which has the most technical writers and technical writing positions, the salary is closer to $55,000. Starting salaries here are in the mid-$40,000 range, which is comparable to the average starting salaries for a research scientist with a Ph.D. but without post-doctoral experience.

  Independent contractors and consultants (freelancers) can make much more than that (hourly rates start at $50 or $60 for experienced writers), but they usually have to pay their own benefits. In general, an experienced technical writer's salary will plateau around $70,000 unless that writer becomes a manager or a freelancer.

- **Job stability:** Technical writing is an expanding field with very good job prospects in many areas of the United States and Canada. It is also a very portable field: you can write almost anywhere that has phone service. Telecommuting is very common.

- **Reasonable hours:** Most writers work from 9:00 to 5:00, give or take half an hour to an hour, and never on weekends unless a deadline makes it absolutely necessary.

- **Equipment:** Each writer has his or her own computer, usually a high-end Macintosh or Windows machine with a large monitor. Our department has two high-speed printers and a scanner. If we are writing about a new machine that the company plans to release, we can borrow that machine if it is small, or we can use one in a lab if it is large. If we are writing about new software, we can get a copy of it to play with.

- **Interpersonal skills:** People skills are more important to a tech writer than to a research scientist because we get information from other people, not from running experiments.

HOW TO BECOME A TECH WRITER

The following list details what worked for me and for other scientists who have successfully made the transition into technical writing:

- Rework your résumé. Most résumés of grad students and post-docs start with a description of their educational background and end with a list of publications with titles that are incomprehensible to anyone outside of the applicant's own subfield. This says "SCIENTIST" in large, bold type.

  Instead, create a functional (skills-based) résumé. Start with a concise job objective, such as "to combine my scientific background and writing skills in a challenging position." List your skills and detail your experience, concentrating on writing and computers. Give brief summaries of your employment experience and education and tell how many times you've been published. Your résumé should be no longer than one or two pages.

- Get some experience. Submit freelance science articles to your local paper. Volunteer to write for or edit the newsletter of the local chapter of the scientific society to which you belong. You need to build up a "portfolio," a body of your work that is not made up only of scientific publications (although successfully funded grant proposals are a plus). Volunteer work is also a good line on a résumé.

- Learn a word processing or desktop publishing program. The more tools of the trade you know, the better. Start with the word processing programs Word or WordPerfect, which most research groups use to write their papers. If you are serious about tech writing, get a copy of FrameMaker, PageMaker, or QuarkXPress, which are desktop publishing programs. Most college bookstores have academic discounts on software. FrameMaker is the most expensive but most useful of the three, and this makes an excellent line on a résumé. Besides, you will need to know one of these programs for your technical writing classes.

- Take technical writing classes. It helps to have a credential on your résumé that does not imply "SCIENTIST." Writing classes are also helpful in learning to write for different audiences, and the classes will "deprogram" you from writing in the dry, passive voice, scientific style. ("A 5-mL aliquot of dichloromethane was added to a round-bottom flask containing compound 1. The mixture was then stirred at ambient temperature for an 8-hour period." Instead clarify who is doing the experiment and say, "Add 5 mL of dichloromethane to compound 1 in a round-bottom flask. Stir at room temperature for 8 hours.")

  The classes are also great for networking. I found my job through a posting in one of my classes. I will probably find my next job through my contacts in other companies, many of whom I met through my classes.

- Check with your local community college or state university campus for technical writing certificate programs. You can take classes part-time while you are still a grad student or post-doc. I started taking classes when I found out that the grant supporting my post-doc position was not renewed (I guess we did not explain the utility of Kb fluorescence spectroscopy well enough). I was tired of research and was going to become a tech writer anyway, but the thought of impending unemployment gave me an incentive to leave research. I kept taking classes after my post-doc ended, and I was out of work for only 2 months when I found my internship.

- Find an internship. Working as an intern can teach you how to be a technical writer in the real world. These jobs are also easier to get than are full-time jobs if you have no experience. Be willing to accept relatively low pay ($8 to $15 per hour) for 3 to 6 months. Internships can lead to a permanent position at the same company or at another company. Either way, you will have marketable experience.

After seeing a posting in one of my classes for an "aspiring tech writer" with scientific experience, I started as an intern. I was lucky to be in the right place at the right time. After 3 weeks as an intern, there was an opening for a full-time writer at my company, and I was hired. I started in February 1996 and was promoted to senior technical writer in January 1997.

Some recruiters will hire inexperienced writers as contractors. This is very useful experience, but be careful to read every word of the contract before you sign. Don't sign just anything because you think you can't find any other job. Also, if you do accept a contract that isn't an internship, don't take less than $20 to $25 per hour for your first job. The average salary for entry-level technical writers/editors in the United States is $43,260.

- Join the Society for Technical Communication (STC). The STC, an international organization of about 15,000 technical writers, is based in Arlington, Virginia. It has chapters in every state in the United States. STC meetings are a great place to network. Each chapter also has a list of available jobs, most of them posted by members or local recruiters. STC contact information is listed at the end of this chapter under Resources. Membership costs $160 per year ($50 for students in technical writing programs).

WHERE TO FIND TECH WRITING JOBS

Most technical writing jobs are not listed in the newspaper. If you don't have many contacts in the tech writing field, then the local STC chapter is the best place to begin your search. College placement offices and technical communication (or English, etc.) departments help their students find jobs. Once you find a job, keep your skills and résumé current. Learn as much as you can about everything. Network as much as you can. You never know what will lead to your next job.

WHERE CAN YOU GO AFTER TECH WRITING?

Most writers eventually become managers of other writers or they become freelancers; that is, they work for themselves as contractors or consultants. They can also go into marketing communications (advertising and public relations work) or science journalism. Some writers prefer to remain as individual contributors at a company, but they move up in rank and pay by changing companies. This is the Silicon Valley way of getting promotions and raises.

Scientists have other career paths. Going back into the lab is an option, but it gets more difficult the longer you are out of the lab. In companies like mine, which are characterized by interdisciplinary teams and a relatively flat (nonhierarchical) organization, lateral moves are common. Research and development scientists often switch research groups or move into process development or marketing. Most marketing people at my company came from the lab bench, as did the executives.

Scientists who are technical writers can also move into areas with more direct customer contact, such as marketing, technical support, sales, and field service. Our company also supports rotations, where you can work in a different area for a month or a few months. I learned a lot by working in our technical support department, taking customer phone calls for a few days, and I plan to do a rotation there for a month later this year.

Outside of industry, the fields of science journalism and science and technology policy are also possibilities because people who work in public policy write many reports.

In short, there are very few limits to what you can do as a technical writer.

RESOURCES

As stated previously, the STC is good for networking and for finding schools with technical writing programs. Membership costs $160 per year ($50 for students in technical writing programs). From its Web site, you can find links to every local chapter that has a Web site. Here is the society's contact information:

Society for Technical Communication
901 N. Stuart St, Suite 904
Arlington, VA 22203-1854
(703) 522-4114
http://stc.org

An excellent reference is *The Tech Writing Game* by Janet Van Wicklen (Facts on File, New York, 1992), ISBN 0-8160-2607-6. It goes into much more depth about the profession than I can here. I highly recommend this book to anyone who might want to become a tech writer.

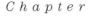

3

SCIENCE WRITING:

Communicating with the Masses

Sue Goetinck Ambrose, Ph.D.
Science Writer, The Dallas Morning News

Thinking about leaving the lab? Do you want sane hours and more variety in your job? Then science writing may be for you. I have been working as a science writer for *The Dallas Morning News* for 10 years, and I feel like I am in college again (only now they are paying me). Every week brings a new topic, and I am learning more about science than ever before. If you are thinking about writing as a career, then you should read this chapter to get a flavor of the field and what training you need to become gainfully employed.

SHOULD YOU BECOME A SCIENCE WRITER?

A personal ad for a scientist who would make a good science writer might go something like this: "BUS (bored, unfulfilled scientist), likes to talk science but hates to do it. I would rather learn a little about many areas of science than spend the rest of my career focused on a single, narrow field. I crave variety. I need to feel like I have accomplished something when I go home for the day. I am willing to leave behind cumbersome, jargon-laden academic prose. I dream of getting published in a matter of a month, a week, or even a few hours. Can you help?"

Absolutely! I have a Ph.D. in molecular genetics. During my 10 years as a science writer with *The Dallas Morning News*, I have met dozens of other writers who have also left the lab. When we talk about how we got into the profession, the reasons are usually the same. Like scientists, we science writers are generally deeply interested in science. We are curious, we love to learn, and we want to make a difference.

But unlike most scientists, those who have become science writers are perfectly happy to observe. In fact, we are downright relieved that we never have to do another experiment. We are so happy being vultures—we can sit and wait until someone else has repeated an experiment 10 times, until they have worked out all the quirks, done all the controls and agonized over a publication. Then, we revel vicariously in their success, write an article about it, and get it in print in a fraction of the time. Doesn't this sound great?

A CHALLENGING FIELD

For me, science writing has been as challenging as it has been satisfying. Although I mainly cover biology issues for the *Morning News*, I have also had the opportunity to write about geology, astronomy, and particle physics. Those were some of the more difficult stories I have done, but what other job would allow me to spend hours on the phone quizzing some of the country's best geologists and physicists about their work? If I were still working as a biologist and wanted to expand my horizons, I would have to settle for reading popular science articles that someone else had written.

Within my primary focus, or "beat," I have covered a huge variety of topics in life sciences—the biology behind mental illness and breast cancer, the cloning of sheep and the genetics of taste, heart development, high blood pressure, immunology, the Human Genome Project, obesity, aging, and many other advances in genetics.

The job is not easy, but it doesn't run me into the ground like research did. This, of course, is because I find reporting and writing a lot more fun.

• •
"The job is not easy, but it does not run me into the ground like research did."
• •

All that said, be forewarned that science writing is not a profession for scientists who just can't come up with a better alternative. If you venture this way, you *will* work hard. Deadlines and editors can be tough. But you will learn a lot, you will reach real people, and (most days, anyway!) you will go home knowing you have accomplished something.

WHO NEEDS SCIENCE WRITERS?

Many groups need science writers. Science writers can be found almost anywhere science is conducted and quite a few places where it is not. From my own unscientific observations, it seems that the most jobs are in a field known as public relations or public information. Virtually every university, medical center, hospital, or institution that does research has its own staff of reporters that keeps tabs on the happenings at the institution. Public information officers, or PIOs for short, write press releases that are distributed to the media, contribute to in-house publications and alumni magazines, and serve as a liaison between reporters and the institution's staff. They also monitor local and national media trends so they know which staff members might have something valuable to say to reporters about the latest hot issue.

Government research institutions, such as the National Institutes of Health or the Department of Energy, also have PIOs, as do many companies with science-related products. And, sometimes, independent public relations firms represent these types of institutions.

Museums or aquariums are another option for science writers. These institutions need writers to publicize research and exhibits, as well as to help design and write signs for the exhibits themselves.

Other outlets include magazines and newspapers (more about newspapers coming up, since that is my focus). There are several popular science magazines—*Discover, Science News, New Scientist, BioScience*, and *Popular Science*, to name a few. Journals such as *Science* and *Nature* have their own reporters, and a lot of general news magazines, such as *Time* and *Newsweek,* also have specialized science writers. Health and trade magazines need writers with a technical background as well.

Some universities, such as Harvard, publish newsletters that summarize the latest advances and trends in a variety of medical specialties. Some of my colleagues have written for children's science books and TV shows. Writers who have been around for a while doing smaller pieces often venture into book writing. One science writer I know uses his writing skills to write speeches and memos for company executives. Another has helped edit an undergraduate biology textbook.

Many people have asked me about freelancing. This is an attractive option for someone who does not want to be tied down to a staff position. A word of caution, though. Most freelancers do not rely on freelance dollars as their sole source of income. Many have part-time jobs or a spouse who helps pay the bills. However, if you get some really good clients, it is possible to survive this way.

So to sum up, there are a lot of different types of jobs for a writer who knows science. But first, you will probably need a little training.

How Do I Become a Science Writer?

After receiving my Ph.D. degree from Washington University in St. Louis, I enrolled in a 9-month science writing program at the University of California, Santa Cruz. In that short time, I learned to write news stories, features, and essays. I got practice reporting and interviewing and did two 10-week internships at *The Californian*, a small paper in Salinas, California. I covered everything from community social programs to murders.

While not all science writers have formal training in journalism, I think it helps. Through the program at Santa Cruz, I met many professional writers and editors who gave me a good sense of the field. And I was able to get those invaluable "clips"—printed newspaper and newsletter articles that served as part of my portfolio when I applied for an internship at the *Morning News*.

There are several programs across the country that train science writers (see end of chapter for more information about how to find these). If you can spare the time and the money, I would recommend applying. The American Association for the Advancement of Science also offers mass media internships every summer. The contacts you will make and the clips you will accumulate will help you get your foot in the door. But if taking one of these programs is not an option, I offer a couple of tips.

First, do whatever it takes to get an article published! Even one clip can get you your next assignment. If you have to write an article for a small newspaper or a newsletter for free, do it! If nothing else, it will give you a flavor for the job. My first clip was a short article that was printed in one of the free community newspapers in St. Louis. I am forever grateful to that paper's editor because my modest clip helped me get into the writing program in Santa Cruz.

• • • • • • • • • • • • • • • • • • • •
"First, do whatever it takes to get an article published! Even one clip can get you your next assignment."
• • • • • • • • • • • • • • • • • • • •

Second, read an introductory undergraduate journalism textbook. This type of book will introduce you to the basics. Even if you do not want to write for a newspaper, the advice in the book should help you get away from academic-style prose and move you toward a writing style that is more easily understood by a layperson. Whatever type of writing is your goal, practicing the newspaper style will teach you to organize your thoughts, to write in a conversational style, and to cut out unnecessary words.

If you do enroll for a journalism or writing program, be prepared to work hard and also to learn a whole new way of thinking. I learned more in my 9 months at Santa Cruz than I did in almost any 9-month stretch working on my dissertation.

WHAT IS A TYPICAL WORK DAY LIKE?

A typical day for me (and probably for most newspaper reporters) starts like this: I get to work around 9:30 A.M. I check my voice mail, my e-mail, and scan my snail-mail to see if there is anything pressing. Then, I read the *Morning News* and look through *The New York Times*. If I have a story in the paper, I check to see how it survived the late-night editing process. What happens next depends on the day of the week and what stories I happen to be working on. Early in the week, I scan "tip sheets," bulletins from the major science journals that summarize what is coming out in that week's issue. I order any scientific papers that look like they might make a good story and save them to "pitch" at the weekly staff meeting. Then I might go to the local university to do an interview, do interviews over the phone, or work on a story. If I have a major story coming out, later in the week I will discuss the text with my editor and the accompanying graphics with the artist. If there is a story that merits "daily" coverage (an article that has to run in the national or local section of the paper the next day), my work day might get a little hectic, especially if sources decide not to call back until an hour before deadline.

Sometimes news will break unexpectedly, such as when NASA scientists reported they had possibly found life on Mars or when Scottish scientists announced that they had cloned a sheep. One morning, when I was still an intern, I lay half asleep and listened to National Public Radio announce that Al Gilman, a Dallas biologist, had won a Nobel prize. Needless to say, that was a busy day!

Big news does not break that often in science, especially compared to beats like crime or politics. So in between interviews and writing, I have time to read journals, press releases, and other publications. Before I started working part-time, I traveled to five or six scientific meetings every year to hear the latest, unpublished research and to meet sources face to face.

IT IS SCIENCE, BUT IS IT NEWS?

One thing I had to adjust to quickly as a newspaper writer is the fact that the science that excites newspaper editors is not always the same as the science that excites scientists. About 90% of the articles that appear in *Science* and *Nature*, for instance, are simply a waste of ink to any newspaper editor. And rightly so. If you are planning to venture into science writing for the public, remember that most people who read your stories, even if they are science buffs, do not care whether a particular enzyme needs magnesium to work. They do care, however, that a sheep has been cloned, and they care about some slightly less startling news too.

As the life sciences reporter at the *Morning News*, it is my responsibility to keep abreast of my beat well enough to know what makes a new development worthy of coverage. Most of the stories I write are my own ideas, but I also get assignments or suggestions from my editors. There is no formula; a lot depends on the publication you write for and the tastes of your editor.

How Do You Explain DNA in Three Sentences?

You shouldn't explain DNA in three sentences. One skill every science writer needs is the ability to explain complicated subjects in just a few words. That means you have to know what to put in and what to leave out. I have written 1500-word articles about genetics without mentioning DNA. "Genetic material," my favorite euphemism for DNA, does just fine in most cases. Sometimes, however, a story calls for a more detailed explanation of DNA. So genetic material becomes "a helical molecule that looks like two springs wound together." A mutation is a "misspelling." I cannot say that "the gene is expressed only in the cone cells of the retina," but I can say that "the gene is turned on only in the cells of the eye that make color vision possible."

And so it goes. When you sit down and write an article about science, you should not tell readers any more than they need to know at that point in the story. Remember that editors also usually have a word limit. For daily newspaper articles, that means putting the meat at the top and saving details for later. Editors generally cut these stories from the bottom. Longer, feature-type articles may have more leeway. With practice, you will get a feel for how much detail you can fit in a story of a given length.

Do Scientists Like Reporters?

Some scientists like reporters, and others do not. Most people I call for stories are happy to talk to me. Generally, they are flattered by the attention, and they think it is important to communicate their research to the public. But occasionally, there are hurdles. The most prominent people in the field, for example, also tend to be the busiest. I once had to schedule a 15-minute phone interview a month in advance.

Other problems include sources who either never call back or call back in a few days, well after the story has appeared in the paper. Rarer, but definitely out there, is the scientist who simply refuses to get on the phone with a reporter. Not much can be done about them, so I do not waste my time trying to convince them.

The biggest worry scientists have is being misquoted. They are used to having control over everything else with their name on it—manuscripts, meeting abstracts, grant applications—and often get nervous when they cannot see the newspaper article before it comes out. Our paper does not allow this preview, and I can usually reassure my sources by telling them that I don't want to be wrong in print any more than they do. If I have questions, I always call them back.

After the article appears, I always send copies to all my sources, whether I ended up quoting them or not. I have found that researchers appreciate this, and if they are the hard-to-reach type, they are more likely to return my calls in the future.

WILL ANYONE READ WHAT YOU WRITE?

If you write a well-written, interesting story, you can bet people will read it. I get feedback from my readers: a couple of letters or phone calls a month is not out of the ordinary. Most have been complimentary, but occasionally I hear from someone who is unhappy with something I wrote, such as one article I did on evolution. A creationist didn't buy what I had written, and he sent me a nasty letter to that effect.

I have also received calls from people who oppose animal research. When I write or call back, I politely explain my reasons for writing the story. There isn't much more to be done—if you write a lot of stories, eventually there will be someone who does not like one.

So that is the life of a newspaper science reporter—never a dull moment! I can't say firsthand what any other science writing job is like day to day because I have only worked at newspapers. But from what I can guess, the general work pace is about the same for someone working at a public information office or a magazine. Each job has its own peculiarities, though, and schedules will vary accordingly.

THE LOGISTICS

Can I Make Money Doing This?

Yes, you can make money in this profession! How much you make depends on where you work. I will give some general salary ranges; these are estimates based on job advertisements and information from friends.

- **Newspapers:** Generally, the bigger the paper, the higher the salary. Small papers (circulation from 25,000 to 40,000) might pay $25,000; experienced reporters at the largest papers might make $70,000 to $100,000 or more in certain cities. Everyone else falls somewhere in between. (Note: Small newspapers generally do not have the resources for a reporter to devote time exclusively to science issues, so he or she will probably cover other beats as well.)

  •
  "Generally, the bigger the paper, the higher the salary."
  •

- **Public information:** Starting salaries can be from $35,000 to $45,000. With more experience and a promotion or two, you might earn $60,000 or more. Large, private institutions or companies are likely to pay more than public institutions.

- **Magazines:** Depending on your experience and ability, starting salaries might be around $30,000. Big-time magazine writers probably make in the $70,000 to $80,000 range.

- **Freelancers:** Fees will depend on the publication. Most freelancers are paid by the word—with word count assigned by the editor. Fees can range anywhere from $0.25 to $2.00 a word and will also vary depending on the publication and the writer's experience. Freelancing is hard work—to earn a steady income, writers need to have several stories going at once, and they need to constantly generate new ideas.

- **Other jobs:** Salaries will vary according to institution and the writer's experience. But in general, science writers can certainly expect to earn at least as much as academic scientists and often more.

How Do I Find a Job?

I see a lot of job advertisements for science writers, so there definitely are jobs to be had. How easy it is to get one obviously depends on your writing and reporting abilities, as well as your own demands. There are more jobs in the cities, and if you are committed to a particular region, your options will be more limited. Job advertisements are posted through the standard institutional channels, and members of the National Association of Science Writers (NASW) can check their Web site for openings. More about NASW later.

What Are My Opportunities for Advancement?

Once you have a job as a science writer, there are several courses your career can take. As you gain experience as a writer, you should be able to get more challenging assignments and to receive promotions and raises. Some writers transfer to more prominent publications when they feel it is time to move on. Others become editors. Last, if you really like writing and don't feel compelled to write about science exclusively, you will have a lot of options. So many people have phobias about writing that organizations will gladly hire someone who can do it without too much effort.

Will I Be Any Good at This?

First of all, you have to like to write. You should enjoy the challenge and have a natural sense of what reads well. Even if you like to write but sometimes struggle or find it hard to get started, don't let that stop you. The more practice you get, the easier it becomes. My writing speed has increased at least by a factor of 10 since I started.

Other Important Qualities

- **Ego:** It shouldn't be big. You cannot be afraid to ask stupid questions, and you cannot afford to get offended when scientists talk down to you. Believe me, some will. Also, be prepared to have your work criticized by editors. The less personally you take their advice, the more you will learn.

- **Self-motivation:** You should have a lot of motivation. Everyone needs encouragement, but you should be able to work independently and take the initiative. This is not usually a problem for someone who has made it through a Ph.D. program.

- **Interpersonal aspects:** You should be able to work well with others. It is important to stay on good terms with your editor. And getting good information from sources requires that you can put them at ease and earn their trust. Do not worry if you have never interviewed anyone before. There are a few tricks that make it a lot easier, and with experience, you will soon become a pro.

- **Accuracy:** This is also a must. You do not want to be wrong in print. You need to have an appreciation for detail and subtlety. And do not misspell anyone's name!

- **Ability to work under pressure:** Feeling the pressure to write fast and on time will come up in almost every writing job I can imagine. Fortunately, writing on deadline also gets easier with practice.

- **An open mind:** This is a given. Unless you are writing fiction or an opinion piece, you have to report what your sources tell you, and it may not be what you expect. You cannot make stuff up or let preconceived notions get in your way. You should be able to ask a lot of questions and listen, listen, listen!

So Is This Better than the Lab?

For me, without question, writing is much better than working in the lab. Becoming a science writer has been a life-saving career move. The only thing I miss about doing research is working with my hands, and that void is easily filled through hobbies. My attention span is too short to be a scientist, so journalism suits me perfectly.

But my new career did take some getting used to. I fill out a time card now and need to be in by a certain time every day. I only get 2 weeks of vacation a year. I cannot wear shorts and a T-shirt to work or take off in the middle of the afternoon for a jog and then return to work all sweaty. My daily stress is a little higher.

But the positives definitely outweigh the negatives. I rarely work weekends or evenings anymore. Also, writing is a field where you can see yourself progressing. Each type of story—short or long, hard news or feature—has its own limitations and possibilities. That means there are elements that you can isolate and improve on. Since leaving the lab, progress has become more obvious and tangible for me.

Last, I have found that my scientific background is more appreciated now than it was when I worked in the lab. If that sounds cheap (I am supposed to be the newspaper's expert in life sciences anyway), then so be it. Having people's respect builds my confidence and makes me feel good about my job.

WHERE CAN I GET MORE INFORMATION?

Check out the National Association of Science Writer's Web page at www.nasw.org. This site will give you more information on the field. (Some links are accessible only to members.) From this site, you can order a book called *A Field Guide for Science Writers*. It is written by prominent science writers and contains more detailed information than I have given here. The back of the book has a list of resources useful to working writers, as well as addresses of university science writing courses programs.

SOME INSPIRATION

If you are reading this book, you are probably already considering leaving the ivory tower. But if you are still having doubts or have a vague sense of guilt, believe me when I say it is okay to leave. When I was considering getting out of basic research, I worried far too much about what other people thought. I wondered if my professors and lab mates thought I had copped out. One professor even tried to reassure me that I really could succeed in research, as if he thought I was taking on a less demanding profession. Even I wondered if I was.

But after making a living as a science writer, I can safely say I did not move to an easier job. Just because science writers write in simple language does not mean the job is simple. If you choose to become a science writer, you can make your career as challenging as you want.

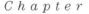

Chapter

4

••••••••••

CREATING A PUBLISHING EMPIRE:

How I Gave up Academia and Became an Entrepreneurial Editor

•••••••••••••••••

An interview with
Roger Longman
Managing Partner, Windhover Information, Inc.

HOW IT ALL STARTED

After finishing my master's degree in English at University of North Carolina-Chapel Hill, I decided I needed a break before plunging onward to the Ph.D. program. My girlfriend and I had always wanted to live in Italy, so I got a job teaching for the University of Maryland's program that provided college courses for U.S. employees (mostly those in the military) posted overseas. I spent about 2 years teaching near Venice and most of a year in Rome before heading back to the United States. While our Italian experience was intellectually and creatively wonderful, we still had a nagging sense of not belonging entirely. We returned to New York City in 1983. My now-wife was a librarian and managed to find employment quickly. I, the failed graduate student, had no job on the near horizon. I decided that I didn't want to go back to school to finish that doctorate—the thought of being a poor student again was less than appealing, and I was not at all sure that scholarship was my destiny. I started looking for a job in the *New York Times* classifieds and was interviewed for many positions, all aimed at things like copyediting or writing.

Alternative Careers in Science

One day, I spotted a mysterious ad for a magazine called *In Vivo* that had no phone number or address, only a post office box to which applications could be sent. I tried to track down its location and could not find anyone who had heard of the magazine. Finally, a librarian acquaintance suggested calling a subscription service; sure enough, it had a listing for *In Vivo* and a phone number. I called the editor and told her I wanted a job with the magazine. She was impressed I had found the office and agreed to an interview.

In Vivo turned out to be owned by Channing,Weinberg, and Company— a prestigious consulting group run by Barry Weinberg and Walter Channing. The group had evolved from a consulting firm, which was then run by John Wilkerson, into a venture capital fund and had decided to publish a health care magazine. For about 6 months I worked on sample articles and was paid per article printed. I then demanded a real, full-time job writing for about 200 subscribers. Meanwhile, the consulting group had split from the venture fund, taking the magazine with it. John Wilkerson became my mentor, teaching me about business consulting and publishing.

I decided that publishing was the field for me. Just as I was getting ready to leave *In Vivo* for a more prestigious position at a national business magazine, my boss stepped down. I became editor, a great situation that lasted for 2 years. By then, John and the other partners were all too well aware that every minute John spent with *In Vivo* added up to unbillable hours! The magazine (like many magazines) lost money all the time, so it was not contributing to the firm's bottom line. By 1986, it was becoming increasingly difficult to manage *In Vivo* as an independent magazine. The reporters wanted to write stories that they thought were interesting and informative, but the consultants wanted stories that would allow their clients to be quoted. Everyone was getting antagonized—the classic tension between editorial and advertising interests.

One of my colleagues, Tucker Swan, had the idea to start listing financing and business development transactions in the biomedical industry in each issue. As we saw the volume of deals, it became obvious we should collect them to create an annual reference book. The first volume of the transactions book sold well (though not quite enough to reach net profit right away), making it clear that folks were interested in the transaction side of health care. This success led us to create an electronic database of the transactions so that we could lay them out on the page in various formats.

The tension between the consulting group and the publishing group got too high for comfort, and John decided to sell the magazine. After several almost-completed deals, I started thinking seriously about taking on the business. A good friend, David Cassak, was unhappy working for what had been his father's publication, *Health Industry Today*, which had been sold to Harper & Row. We had many discussions about working together and convinced each other that this was the opportunity. Our plan was to buy 20% of the company, leaving Wilkerson with 40% and finding a minority partner to buy the remaining 40%. But we couldn't persuade anyone to take on that final 40%.

In the end, my brother and David's dad decided to help us out financially. Negotiations were long and difficult, but we ended up owning 90%, with Wilkerson keeping a 10% stake, which we bought out a few years later.

ON OUR OWN

In Vivo and the deals database became officially ours in September 1989. We named the new company Windhover Information, after a favorite poem of ours, and moved the business to Connecticut. The entire team consisted of myself, David, and two other full-time folks (who, amazingly, are still here). The first year was excruciating—we had no business or marketing experience and needed to jack the subscriber level over the existing 200 if we were to have a chance of breaking even, much less making money.

By the second year, things started to turn around. We never really became marketing wizards, but in 1990, the biomedical industries were becoming strong forces in the stock market. Thanks to that higher profile, the readers—potential investors and corporate partners—came across us in their search for information, and we actually broke even! By the next year, we turned a profit. We learned two big lessons from this experience: you can learn by doing (though it can be painful), and timing is everything.

Our business began to evolve as we learned more about the information needs of our growing readership. We became more involved with tracking transactions and began publishing information about pharmaceutical strategic alliances. This change brought in more cash, which allowed us to host a conference about deal making. In 1991, our first Pharmaceutical Strategic Alliances Conference was a big hit and, since then, has been held in New York every year.

•••••••••••••••••••••
"Our business began to evolve as we learned more about the information needs of our growing readership."
•••••••••••••••••••••••

I started giving speeches at conferences organized by other groups, and *In Vivo* continued publishing analytical articles that no other company was covering. David and I hold our reporters to a very high standard. We are convinced that it is critical for the pieces to provide a new way of looking at industry issues, in a format that will appeal to the smartest people in the industry.

We made the database more sophisticated and began selling it electronically by the mid-1990s. In 1996, we launched *Start-Up: Windhover's*

Review of Emerging Medical Ventures, which focused on the venture capital side of the device, biopharmaceutical, and diagnostics industries. By addressing different industry segments, the firm again expanded its potential subscriber base.

As the transaction database became more sophisticated in the late 1990s, it also became a significant revenue generator for us. We began to expand our conference business, starting a EuroBiotech Conference to introduce U.S. biotech companies to mid-size European firms. This was a financial failure the first few years until the market caught up in the third year and U.S./mid-size European deals suddenly became in vogue. It has been 10 years, and this conference is still going strong. And we have added three other conferences to our growing list.

In 2004, we took on some investors and made our first acquisition— Medtech Insight, an information company in California focused on the medical device industry. It brought us a fast-growing newsletter, a market research reports business, a series of conferences, and about 15 new employees.

A Typical Day

Just as our business has evolved, my job within that business has evolved. Windhover employs about 10 writers today, so much of my time is spent working on story ideas, editing, talking to writers, and talking on the phone with people in the industry about current issues. I also still write articles every month.

A key part of my job now is looking for ways to improve our products or to create new products that customers will be willing to pay for. I have to stay in touch with the health care market to do this well. One great way of keeping contact has been speaking regularly at industry events in the United States and abroad. This has given me the chance to let potential clients get a sense of the expertise within our firm, hopefully enticing them to become paying customers. I am also often invited to talk to pharmaceutical company management groups about strategic issues.

In the early days, David handled much of the financial and marketing sides of the business, while I headed up editorial and policy aspects. Today, we have a COO who manages the commercial side of the company and many of the day-to-day details. Our board of directors is also extremely helpful. Our chairman, Norman Selby, built McKinsey's pharmaceutical practice, worked in top management at Citigroup, and was CEO of a biotech company. Another board member, Vaughn Kailian, was a pharmaceutical marketing executive, was CEO of Cor Therapeutics, and then became vice chairman of Millennium Pharmaceuticals.

The Best Parts of the Job

My favorite parts of the job are getting out and talking to people in different sectors of the industry, finding out what is going on in companies throughout a sector, learning about intriguing strategies and projects that are underway, and trying to understand what led to the creation of those strategies. Essentially, I get paid to get an insider's view of the top issues and trends affecting the industry from the most creative, intelligent people creating those strategies and trends.

"Essentially, I get paid to get an insider's view of the top issues and trends affecting the industry from the most creative, intelligent people creating those strategies and trends."

The central paradox of the stories I report is that there are strategies you can learn and models you can follow, but every situation is so different that you really can't follow models blindly. Think of this as trying to understand the broad principles to apply fluidly to your company's specific situation. As a writer, I have to understand enough of those specific details to understand the story, but I then must be able to talk about how to generalize these so they apply to a reader's specific company situation.

Two important ingredients are needed to do this job well:

- The ability to write reasonably well—it turns out that you don't have to be the best, but you do need some basic skills (and a great editor)
- The ability to analyze business situations and come up with interesting perspectives on business topics

This combination makes for a rare entity. There are many great writers who can't analyze and great analysts who can't write worth a damn. To be in an editorial position at any level, you need a strong streak of curiosity to fuel the pursuit of interesting stories. You need to be willing to track down and talk to strangers and not be intimidated by highfalutin titles.

For publications such as *In Vivo*, it is crucial to have a strong desire to be truly thoughtful about a specific issue. The articles we want to publish require a writer to be creatively analytical, not superficial, and to be willing to make the leap from analysis to hypothesis. When looking at the world where business and science intersect, the "ultimate" truth is just too difficult to track down.

"The articles we want to publish require a writer to be creatively analytical, not superficial, and to be willing to make the leap from analysis to hypothesis."

What is more important for our readers is to have an interesting and defensible position, to raise interesting ideas that are inherently reasonable.

What won't work: shyness, stodgy thinking, needing someone else to give you the answer. Be willing to take a chance—even if you are wrong, you are raising interesting issues to consider.

So How Do You Get This Job?

First, to get a job in editorial/publishing, you have to do your homework—research the key publications in the sector you want to cover, read several issues of each to get a sense of their style, talk to subscribers to learn what makes these publications admirable, and then contact the publisher!

A great way to get your foot in the door is to contribute strong articles to key publications as a freelancer. Talk to the smartest people you can find in the area on which you want to report; then find out what intriguing stories they would like to read and identify an unusual take on an important issue for your chosen sector. With this idea outline in hand, approach one of the publications and pitch that story! Publications usually are willing to pay a relatively small sum for freelance work, which gives you a chance to show the publisher your capabilities with a real example of your work.

What Does Publishing Pay?

Pay levels vary widely depending on the specific job description, your level of experience and popularity with the target audience, and the publication. The pay scale is tied somewhat to the revenue-generating capabilities of the publications.

Most publishing companies make their money primarily from advertising, with some contribution from subscription fees. The rates that can be charged for ads are based on the number of subscribers and the "quality" of those readers. Quality is the ability of the readers to buy the services of the advertisers—the more revenue generated by the ads, the better the quality of the readership for those advertisers.

In the case of Windhover, we make nearly all of our money on the sales of our information—through our subscriptions, database, conference attendance, and report fees. Local publications (e.g., *San Francisco Chronicle*) and trade press (e.g., *Genetic Engineering News*) tend to pay lower salaries than national business publications (e.g., *Business Week*, *Wall Street Journal*). A columnist whose articles are highly regarded and draw strong reader response can negotiate for better pay than a local beat reporter.

Editor positions start at around $40,000 and can get as high as $80,000, though significant seniority usually is needed to get past the $60,000 mark.

Publishers typically are paid in the higher end of the range and often participate in profit-sharing plans.

WHAT IS NEXT IN MY CAREER PATH?

It would be pretty tough to beat my current job. While I am talking to you, I am in jeans, I have no boss, and I can call anybody at any biomedical company and pick their brains. I can speak or write about my opinions without fear that this will dramatically shorten my career. Windhover has a staff of 50 great folks who are very smart and fun to work around. I've had the chance to make many friends in the industry with whom I can sit around and brainstorm about new opportunities.

While I am pretty happy with my job description these days, it would be nice not to work quite so hard. Because of my editorial responsibilities, I can't take seats on boards of directors, and I can't invest in stocks in the sector I know the most about because of conflicts of interest. If things do change in the next 5 years, I would like to work less and focus more on music, tennis, and learning other languages.

Chapter

5

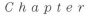

BUSINESS INFORMATION SERVICES:

Providing the Data for Industry

•••••••••••••••••

Mark D. Dibner, Ph.D., M.B.A.
President, BioAbility, LLC

I could not have planned my career in advance because the biotechnology industry did not exist when I was getting my undergraduate degree, and it was just barely getting off the ground when I completed my Ph.D. degree. I thought I was going to wind up as an academic scientist for life. Instead, I wound up in a large corporation, and the evening M.B.A. program I thought I was going to hate actually turned out to be enjoyable. An opportunity I never expected materialized, causing me to leave the research lab for good to enter a career in business information nearly 20 years ago. Today, I have two "professions" that I work at each day—I am in the information business and I am an entrepreneur.

HOW MY PATH CHANGED DIRECTION

I was always sure that I would end up as a physician—it was my goal. In high school, I took all the science classes I could cram into my schedule. In a pre-med program at the University of Pennsylvania I continued on the science path—with one twist. As a physiological psychology major I was able to conduct my own bench research. I liked that. After my tenth-or-so rodent experiment, I was hooked and more interested in research than in a straight medical school program.

Next, I found myself in New York City, at Cornell Medical School, in a Ph.D. program in Neurobiology and Behavior. My research was in developmental neurobiology with a minor focus in pharmacology. I took the basic science courses with the medical students and spent the rest of my time in the lab, while they spent their in the clinic. It reinforced my focus on the research pathway, rather than the life of a physician.

Completing the Ph.D. provided some important contributions to my life. First, it represented a focused and original body of work that I took to a logical conclusion. Few people work on a major, multi-year project with real end points. Second, it taught me to think using the scientific method, where no statement can be made if not supported by fact or testable theory. Third, it taught me how to write. Dr. Ira Black, my Ph.D. advisor, took it upon himself to teach me how to write well with clarity of thought. All three were important lessons that have proven valuable in my career.

Subsequent to graduate school, I completed two post-docs in Denver and San Diego—totaling four years. I was on the way to becoming a life-long academic research scientist, but fate took me on another turn. In applying for academic jobs, I was contacted by a major corporation that promised me the ability to do basic research without hindrance and without ever having to write a grant proposal. On top of that, the salary was about 20–25% higher that the universities were offering. Therefore, I signed on board at E.I. du Pont in Wilmington, Delaware.

In my 6 years at Du Pont (1980 to 1986), I was able to do good research. One of the highlights was that, after only 1 year there, they allowed me to do a 4-month sabbatical in Cambridge, England, at Leslie Iversen's laboratory, following in my Ph.D. advisor's footsteps and working with some bright young scientists. Other skills were picked up in industry, especially an appreciation and understanding of intellectual property, some personnel management skills related to the two or three employees who worked in my lab, some human resource skills needed during the interview and hiring process, and an understanding of how to work within—and sometimes around—a large bureaucracy.

After 2 years at Du Pont, I found out that the company would pay for advanced coursework if it related to my job. Du Pont took a broad view of related coursework and preferred it to be related to a degree program, not just isolated courses. This generally meant getting a law degree or an M.B.A. I was

"I knew I wouldn't like law school, and I had no interest in business. But the M.B.A. program was the lesser of two evils."

single at the time and had liked school in the past, so I wanted to spend some of my evenings doing something. I knew I wouldn't like law school, and I had no interest in business. But the M.B.A. program was the lesser of two evils. I enrolled in Widener University in 1983 for their evening M.B.A. program.

Since I did not think I would like business school, I decided my first course should be the one I was convinced I would hate the most. The plan was to hate the course so much I would get this coursework idea out of my system and drop out. Good plan. So, I took a class in managerial accounting. I did not know a debit from a credit (still don't) and felt it was time to learn this. It turns out that this course was, in fact, about strategic decision making. It included two of the most useful concepts I learned during the M.B.A. program—sunk costs and opportunity costs. I actually liked business school!

I stayed with the M.B.A. program for the ensuing 2½ years. I was doing good, but not earth-shattering, research at Du Pont while finding I enjoyed learning about strategic planning. Widener also had a requirement that would drastically alter my career—it required a master's thesis of all M.B.A. students. I chose to write about the impact of biotechnology on the pharmaceutical industry.

Being someone who pursued a Ph.D., I wasn't about to write a thesis-length paper without publishing it. I had created two databases, one on U.S. biotechnology companies and one on the actions and alliances that biotechnology companies were forming worldwide, as part of my background work for the thesis. I published two papers on the advent of the U.S. biotechnology industry.

Stuff happened. Good stuff. The editor of *Science* phoned and asked me if I would write a lead article on the fledgling biotechnology industry. A manager at the National Science Foundation (NSF) phoned and asked me if the foundation could give me a grant to conduct further research on the industry to be used as part of their upcoming Science Indicators Report. The head of the management and technology program at the Wharton School asked if he could make me a Fellow of the Wharton School and if I would work with him in studying the biotechnology industry. To top it all off, the Western Pharmaceutical Society called and asked if they could sponsor my travel to Banff, Canada for a week, so I could present the keynote address at their annual international meeting.

Something was happening here. I was a good scientist—perhaps very good—but I had never been asked to give a keynote lecture, write a lead article in *Science*, or be given money by the NSF. So that November I sat down and asked myself the answer to this question—If I could create a job that would be exactly what I wanted to do, what would it be? In my answer to myself, I described creating a group that would study the biotechnology industry and provide strategic business information. This group would have three main resources—the databases I had begun for my M.B.A. thesis, a good library of resources specific to commercial biotechnology, and staff who focused only on commercial biotechnology. Given enough time and financial support to build these resources, I suggested that the group could provide strategic information services for a fee.

The next step was to use the miracle of word processing to take this virtual job description and turn it into a letter. I had interviewed a new type of organization—biotechnology centers—for my *Science* article. In 1985, there were only two centers of any repute, the Maryland Biotechnology Institute and the North Carolina Biotechnology Center (NCBC).

I wrote a letter to each, telling them that if they would invest in me and my biotechnology information program as a new division of their centers, then the program would bring them international attention, provide a great resource to the community they serve, and ultimately bring in some funding for the research we could do with the possibility of someday becoming self-sufficient. As it turns out, the Maryland Biotechnology Institute was mostly a result of creative publicity at the time, but NCBC was real and very eager to talk. The organization had only eight employees at the time and more money than it could spend. Timing is everything.

We talked, my wife and I moved to Durham, and the Biotechnology Information Program was born at NCBC. I left for-profit, large industry for a small, state-funded, private, not-for-profit organization. In retrospect, all of the things I put in my letter selling the program to NCBC have come to pass—and more. The program evolved into the Institute for Biotechnology Information (IBI) in 1992 to give it an aura of a separate entity, even though it was still a division of the center. I was director of IBI and a vice president of the center.

We had nine employees at IBI and an international reputation. The databases grew tremendously, and we sold them. We collected data and published them as directories. We were asked by companies to do special studies for them. And we were asked to serve as government contractors and subcontractors to complete studies. The library had grown to be what was arguably the best public library in the world for commercial biotechnology. The biotechnology center got the attention it sought, along with some income, and was able to provide a tremendous resource to the community it served.

While at NCBC, I was able to pursue four other things I enjoy very much. First, I was able to teach. As another example of timing, my moving to North Carolina coincided with the firing of a nonproductive faculty member of Duke University's Fuqua School of Business. I met with the dean to see if I could teach perhaps an occasional lecture and walked out as an adjunct associate professor teaching one or two courses each year in management of technology and, more recently, in entrepreneurship. I was with Duke for 13 years. I had previously taught courses in Denver and San Diego during my post-doctoral positions but had never taught graduate students. My fellowship at Wharton and my lead articles in *Science* led them to believe I knew what I was doing.

The second thing I was able to do at NCBC was to continue to write and publish. While there, I authored four books, two on U.S. biotechnology and two on Japanese biotechnology. We were doing numerous studies, and I was able to publish about 50 papers during those years, mostly on commercial biotechnology. Working for NCBC, I did not have to account for my hours to be financially productive, so I could take the studies we were doing and follow through with published articles.

The third thing I liked to do was to travel and make presentations about my work. I lectured about 10 to 15 times each year at a national or international venue. I enjoy lecturing, and it helped me spread the word about our work to thousands of people each year. Like publishing, it was a form of free marketing, and getting out and about was great for networking.

Networking is the fourth important skill I was able to build during my years at NCBC. My boss, Dr. Charles Hamner, president of NCBC, was an excellent mentor. He was happy to have us spread the word about NCBC at meetings, with societies, wherever. I joined the Board of Directors of the Association of Biotechnology Companies. I founded the National Council of Biotechnology Centers and served as its chairman; I got involved with the Drug Information Association, running the biotechnology track at their annual meeting; I gave keynote lectures to countless societies and groups; I served on national research council working groups; I was on three editorial boards of industry journals; and I was on the boards of directors of two companies. I networked.

During my 8 years at NCBC, our IBI group also grew and established many ties. We worked for an increasing number of clients. We created more than 20 published books and directories. We were quoted frequently. Our abilities to do market research, competitor analysis, technology assessments, international studies, and a panoply of special research projects grew. This was a team effort of people with great abilities.

It was nice working for someone who was supportive and nurturing, as both the Center and Dr. Hamner were. But IBI was growing into its own entity and approaching self-sufficiency. The state legislature also realized this and saw that NCBC had a division that was actually bringing in money.

At the beginning of 1993, the state gave Dr. Hamner a mandate to make IBI self-sufficient within 5 years. He, in turn, gave me 3 years to accomplish this goal. We talked and agreed that if he gave me a year to plan and prepare, I would take IBI as a private, for-profit company. This had benefits all around—the center got to beat the mandate from the legislature by 4 years, and it got to spin off a company for the first time, which would help satisfy its mandate of creating jobs and revenues related to biotechnology. I had confidence that IBI could succeed as a company. I was ready to become an entrepreneur.

ENTREPRENEURSHIP

The Institute for Biotechnology Information, LLC, was launched in July 1994 as a new company owned by my wife and myself (and financed through remortgaging our house). We took three people from our group at NCBC and hired two others to begin the new company. A contract was drafted giving IBI 3 years of work from NCBC to continue to provide some of the information services we had been supplying internally. We had to leave the library behind because it was a showplace and attracted considerable attention. But the center was bound to maintain the library for 5 years and could not compete in providing information services for profit for that time. IBI moved to new, modest digs nearby in Research Triangle Park.

IBI provided strategic business information in biotechnology and pharmaceuticals to a wide variety of clients, from government agencies to biotechnology firms to large corporations. About one-fifth of our income came from sales of products—four books, a monthly journal, and our databases (if the reader is interested, details can be found at www.bioability.com).

Four-fifths of our income came from special studies, which varied widely in nature and scope. For example, at the time of this writing, we have now been in business for 10 years, and our active projects include writing two business plans—one for a scientist with a new separations technology who is funding a new company out of his life savings, and one for a group within a billion-dollar corporation that wants to spin off its technology to form a new diagnostics company. We are also conducting a survey about needs in biodefense; helping a granting authority evaluate the commercial potential of grant proposals; assisting some investors with deep due diligence for a potential investment; and setting up an international data collection study. In addition, we are writing four books to be published by *BioWorld Today*—three on venture capital sources and one on markets for biodefense products.

IBI grew in its first 3 years from 6 to 14 employees. We were growing slowly but steadily. The three strengths we have are our resources, such as internal and external books and databases, our reputation and networking, and our people. IBI was created to be a team of people with complementary skills who could work well as a team. The majority of our staff has advanced graduate degrees. Three of us have Ph.D.s, two have M.B.A.s, and others have an assortment of masters degrees.

What we provide, in a nutshell, is strategic business information. The main strengths we bring are the strengths I described that I learned throughout my career. These skills are the ability to design scientific research, the ability to write and edit, the ability to teach (clients), and the ability to network for both new business development and information gathering.

With the excellent level of personnel availability in the Research Triangle Park area of North Carolina, we could fill most of our positions with candidates who already had Ph.D.s. In actuality, only the research jobs really benefit from a Ph.D. background, so we make efforts to not hire those with Ph.D.s for positions in which they would be overqualified (and never satisfied). Within IBI, the employee with a Ph.D. is useful in data gathering, report writing, explaining scientific know-how for a variety of studies we do, and analyzing and assessing data.

In 1998, sensing the potential explosion in the field of pharmacoeconomics, I started a second company, Strategic Outcomes Services (SOS). For this, I partnered with the former worldwide director of pharmacoeconomics at Glaxo Wellcome (and the person who coined the term *pharmacoeconomics* many years before). During its 3 years, this company grew from 3 people to 18, and I was president of both IBI and SOS for most of that time. To save my marriage, I gave up teaching at Duke.

I would not recommend running two organizations simultaneously—too much confusion, and when the phone rings you never know which hat you are supposed to be wearing. During SOS's 3 years in business, we purchased a small but well-known consulting firm and grew our business dramatically. Thankfully for me, after 3 years, a public company, CareScience, offered to buy us and we accepted. I was back to one hat, and in January 2001, we simultaneously sold SOS and changed the name of IBI to BioAbility. We chose the name BioAbility because in actuality, we were neither an institute nor were we just focused on biotechnology.

I learned three very important lessons from my SOS experience. The first is that I liked starting companies. It is what I like to do the most. It finally struck me that I am an entrepreneur. The second is that, mostly by luck, I picked as my major partner someone whom I liked, respected, and with whom I saw eye-to-eye on most issues. This connection kept us together in the first year when times were tough and allowed us to handle the sale of our joint business successfully. The third lesson, a dark one, was something new to me. When money is on the table, people can get ugly. When we went to sell, some of our minority partners fussed and became, well, child-like. They did and said some mean-spirited things and made accusations that were astounding.

But I was done with SOS, had a little change in my pocket, and enjoying running BioAbility.

We are about to celebrate our eleventh anniversary as a company. The team is smaller, having weathered the tumultuous period between 2001 and 2004. The year 2003 almost did us in, but we survived. We are still a team and doing much of the same work we have done all along.

Looking back at the 28 years since receiving my Ph.D. and my 11 years as a business owner, I realize that a lot has happened. I am the author or coauthor of 10 books and have published over 110 papers, more than 80 of which came out after my M.B.A. and have a technology/business flare. I have started three companies, taught many students, and perhaps most astounding, have kept and grown a family and am still in business. Over the years, I have written about 15 business plans and contributed to countless others.

One thing I have tried to instill in others around me (with limited success) is to give back to the profession. During the last 19 years, I have been on four editorial boards and six company and organization boards of directors; have chaired committees for professional societies; and have assisted dozens of students and others with their careers. Moreover, I have hosted a luncheon for local life science company presidents for 10 years now—a great networking group. None of these things had associated remuneration, but all were to help others in my profession. In turn, with the networking and friendships, they served to help me, I am sure. I see too many people with Ph.D.s in jobs, as employees, but not really building a career—a shame.

I have one other related story to tell . . . nothing to do with my science Ph.D. but a lot to do with my career as an entrepreneur. In 2003, my son (then 13) and I taught ourselves to build a computer. We liked the process so much that we decided to build, or refurbish, older computers and give them to kids who cannot afford computers. Because it was 2003, there was less work at BioAbility than I would have liked to have had, but at least I had plenty of time to work on this project with my son. Thus, Kramden for Kids was formed. We donated computer systems to 35 families, plus we gave another 15 computers to the school—all the computers were fixed in our basement. At the end of the year, every honor roll student at Brogden Middle School in Durham, North Carolina, had a computer in their home.

Kramden for Kids was incorporated in late 2003, and our 501(c)3 not-for-profit charitable status was attained in 2004. We are now seeking funds to take this project out of our basement and into real office space with a paid director so that every honor roll student in all 10 middle schools in Durham will have a computer in their home next year . . . and other cities after that. Dozens of people have offered to support the project with their time and money.

While I am proud of BioAbility, I am equally proud of Kramden, Inc. (see www.kramden.org). Social entrepreneurship is a growing movement in the United States, and the knowledge that you can trade time for a social good, like closing the technology gap or saving the environment from computers discarded before their time, is a wonderful high. But I realize that the entrepreneurial bent that I learned through BioAbility and SOS is the same for the charitable sector.

WHERE THE TIME GOES

Because I have two jobs—running a small but growing business and working in the information business—my day is almost equally divided between the two. Half of my time is spent nurturing and growing the business. A wide variety of tasks is devoted to maintaining the business. I work on personnel issues, marketing, quality assurance, financial issues, and many other business functions. I cannot leave out managing.

The most important statement on managing is also the simplest. As Harold Geneen, the CEO of ITT put it, "Managers must manage." If you realize that the buck stops here and are willing to make the decisions necessary to keep things running, that is half the battle. But the other half is that management decisions need to be made, and you cannot abdicate this responsibility. Of course, early on in a new company, much time is spent making some pretty mundane decisions—choosing insurance, telephone systems, copiers, software packages, printers, and other such things. Considerable time is also spent with a variety of service providers, such as attorneys, accountants, and others.

• •
"The most important statement on managing is also the simplest. As Harold Geneen, the CEO of ITT put it, 'Managers must manage.'"
• •

The task I enjoy second most surprises me. I am involved in all areas of marketing for BioAbility. This is mostly because potential clients have seen me lecture, have read one of my books or papers, or have been told to contact me. I am trying to change this, but to date, most new work comes directly through me. I enjoy talking with prospective clients, preparing proposals, and reeling them in.

My other job, as an information provider, is equally challenging. BioAbility has an excellent staff, and we work well as a team, but I have my own role on the team. My areas of expertise, in strategic planning, regional development, and international competitiveness in biotechnology, require that I take the lead in some of BioAbility's studies. For example, we were hired to do projects for the states of Connecticut and Rhode Island to assist with their local development of biotechnology. In other cases, I am specifically requested to work on a business plan. Finally, I like to serve as quality control for our studies, doing a final check and edit of all reports that go out.

I typically work long hours, but on my own terms. I have a wonderful and understanding spouse—no entrepreneur should be without one—and a growing son. I work full days, weekdays, but try to get home to my family at a reasonable hour. When the family goes to bed, I stay up and work an additional 2 to 4 hours. I am a night owl and do my best work late at night, so I can spend a good amount of time with family, I can coach soccer or take Tae Kwon Do with my son, and I can still put in the 55 to 65 hours it takes to run a business and get the work done. What does keep me away from the family is the travel. I typically go somewhere one or two times each month.

WHERE BIOABILITY IS GOING

While BioAbility has grown its customer base, it no longer looks to build a larger staff. About 6 years ago, I had predicted that the staff would grow to 20 to 25 employees. We are currently at 9 and plan to stay in the 9 to 12 range. There are two reasons for this. The first is the availability of many scientists who can aid us on specific projects or in other consulting firms that can partner with us on projects. This way, we can keep our head count low but still provide a vast amount of expertise.

The second reason is less positive. Not only has the economy been rough on our clients, and therefore us, but the advent of the Internet and common use of search engines has cut into our business. Because we estimate that someone can get 40% of any answer through simple Internet searches (e.g., through Google), many feel they can get what they need from one of these research engines and, therefore, don't think it is necessary to hire an information provider. Luckily, more people realize that their ability to gather accurate and complete information is limited without extra resources, and we can still remain in business helping these clients. We have augmented our offerings by writing more business plans and helping more regions develop their life sciences community. But the old business model, per se, is dead.

Getting into the Business

We have a variety of jobs at BioAbility, but the one most relevant to a graduate with a Ph.D. in science is on our research team. We seek people with strong research backgrounds who have made the decision to leave the lab. A strong and broad understanding of research and the biological sciences is required. Also required are an excellent telephone presence for the telephone interviews for primary data collection; excellent writing and editing skills; advanced use of word processing, spreadsheet, and database programs; some statistical and analytical background; and great teamwork. Desired, but not usually available, is a background with business issues and concepts. The business aspects usually are learned on the job.

Two of BioAbility's researchers hold Ph.D.s. One has a background in plant agricultural biotechnology, but she has headed dozens of research projects for us in fields from pharmaceuticals to international assessments in her 6 years with BioAbility. The other has a Ph.D. in bioengineering, and she, too, has worked on a wide variety of projects. The other important attribute for a researcher in this area is a high degree of flexibility. We never know who will hire us to research what from one week to the next.

Paths to This Career

Large corporations often have many employees involved in competitive intelligence or in strategic information. Many of these employees come from the research ranks within the company. Other companies, such as venture capital firms or investment houses, need people with scientific training to assess proposals, markets, and competition to make sound investment decisions.

Unfortunately, most scientists with Ph.D.s do not have the business background necessary to work in these areas, and they don't tend to have any sort of formal information training. With Internet searches becoming more ubiquitous, however, this training may be obtained on *a de facto* basis. The business training can be received on the job if the work environment is conducive to this.

Not many companies like BioAbility exist, but there are some large consulting companies, such as KPMG Peat Marwick or Ernst and Young, that would hire researchers with Ph.D.s to do business studies. An understanding of business would be helpful, and it can come from experience in industry or even from an added M.B.A.

CONCLUDING THOUGHTS

I could not have chosen this career path if I had tried. Paying attention to unexpected opportunities was important. I enjoy all aspects of the current phase of my career, from the entrepreneurial pressures to managerial requirements. I have a constant sense of being challenged and a constant sense of having a growing and highly satisfying career. The work always takes exciting twists; we get new research projects weekly, and we have the chance to learn about many fascinating subjects. The studies we do become good fodder for writing papers and lecturing, both of which I enjoy. Most of all, when we see that our market research or business plan results in getting needed funding for an entrepreneur or when we pull together information that is used to further commercial biotechnology in a state, the personal satisfaction is tremendous.

·········

THE FINANCIAL WORLD

··················

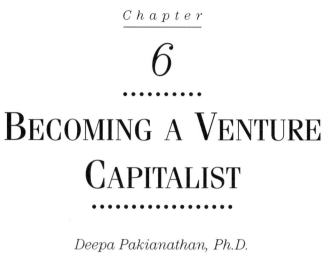

Chapter

6

· · · · · · · · · ·

BECOMING A VENTURE CAPITALIST

· · · · · · · · · · · · · · ·

Deepa Pakianathan, Ph.D.
Partner, Delphi Bioventures

STARTING IN THE LAB

I finished my Ph.D. in immunology in 1993. For a large part of 1992, I combed through the back of *Science* magazine reading the want ads for post-doctoral positions. I was at the time becoming a little disillusioned with academic science. I thought that the scientific questions we asked were interesting but did not impact our understanding of disease in a way that would lead to new therapeutic options. The balance was tipped for good when I met Carol Nacy at an immunoparasitology conference. We had an eye-opening conversation about post-docs in the industry that convinced me to give working for the industry a shot. Carol at the time was at Walter Reed but subsequently moved to EntreMed, Inc., and then cofounded Sequella. Carol was instrumental in introducing me to scientists at Genentech Inc., Immunex, Inc., and Genetics Institute, Inc., and helping me decide to accept the Genentech post-doc offer. This decision was clearly the right one for my future career in venture capital, as seen in retrospect. I am still amazed that every decision I have made since then has been the "right" career choice.

Alternative Careers in Science
Copyright © 2006 Elsevier Inc. All rights reserved.   **61**

The post-doc at Genentech taught me a lot about drug discovery and drug development, even though most of my research did not directly impact those areas. There was a lot to learn, and you had to be pretty proactive about attending seminars in areas other than your little niche of research. Genentech is very academic in some of its approaches. All scientists have to present their work to a group of peers on a regular schedule. You could learn all about process science, preclinical animal models, and clinical statistical analysis if you wanted. There was also an impressive list of people from the outside world who were invited to Genentech to give seminars.

GETTING A TASTE FOR BUSINESS AND FINANCE

As far as career options went, a post-doc at Genentech in the mid-1990s was encouraged to pursue jobs in biotech—preferably at companies other than Genentech. The obvious reason being that there were few job openings at Genentech, and the chances of one of them being open at the time while looking for a job were slim to none. So this post-doc dutifully went off and interviewed for several scientist jobs at companies that shall remain nameless (because the jobs turned out to be less than exciting and seemed at the time to be rather dead-end career choices).

There were other factors that helped me decide to seek a career outside the lab. Genentech had exposed me to very powerful positive and negative examples of mentoring and career choices. I also had spent a fair amount of time trying to put together a company around a molecule that Genentech wanted to out-license. The molecule in question had been on a development path—it worked in animal models and was slated to go into preclinical development toxicology studies. However, there was not a clear choice for realistic clinical studies, and Genentech decided not to move forward but rather out-license the molecule.

A couple of us decided to see if we could put together the necessary resources to license it ourselves and develop it within a new company. This included outsourced manufacturing, collaborations for additional animal models, and possible funding—my first real view of venture capital. My job was to price and source possible manufacturers. The business and entrepreneurial aspects of that little project clearly interested me more than the next experiment done in triplicate and repeated four times.

The easy choice would have been to go back to school and get an M.B.A. degree, which was not palatable after 5 years in graduate school. So I chose the hard way. Now don't get me wrong: I love science and, most of all, I love biology. So a nonlaboratory career *had* to involve science.

The choices, after speaking to a lot of people, were whittled down to management consulting, investment banking, venture capital, mutual fund/

buy-side, and business development. That is when the hard work and the growth of a thick skin began. I called everyone I knew. There were several people who just did not return phone calls or who gave me the brusque brush-off, but I was surprised by how helpful the majority of people were. The two who were the most helpful were David Ebersman and Rod Ferguson, both of whom were in the business development group at Genentech. They opened their contact databases and made a lot of introductions for me, particularly in the investment banking and venture capital worlds. Another person who helped me a lot was Leo Hopf, a management consultant who was married to the daughter of one of my graduate school professors.

Breaking into the Bank

Through these three contacts, I was introduced to a number of key people in each of the chosen areas of interest. My choices were quickly whittled down. At the time, venture funds simply did not hire post-docs, unlike the present, when those with Ph.D.s and M.D.s fresh out of training are being hired as associates. Every venture capitalist (VC) fund gave me a quick "no." Management consulting seemed like the most obvious choice since those firms were used to hiring candidates with Ph.D.s, especially the big ones like McKinsey. However, I was limited to choosing west coast jobs, so the big firms were out. Leo Hopt came through for me and introduced me to his partners who did pharmaceutical and biotech work. This is where I flunked out since I did not have the requisite financial knowledge that their firm wanted. I had taken one introductory finance class at San Francisco State, but that clearly was not enough. I was competing against a base of financial knowledge garnered by those with M.B.A.s.

Interestingly enough, there was a fair amount of interest from the investment banks in hiring a person with a Ph.D. as a research analyst. At the time, there were a few people with Ph.D.s on Wall Street but not anywhere near the number that there are today. Again, these introductions came through Rod Ferguson and David Ebersman at Genentech. Timing and luck were on my side this time. I was offered a job as a research associate with a senior research analyst at a boutique investment bank, Genesis Merchant Group. The investment bank was looking for someone with a broad scientific knowledge and industry experience that would complement the financial skills of the senior research analyst. My Ph.D. and

"The investment bank was looking for someone with a broad scientific knowledge and industry experience that would complement the financial skills of the senior research analyst."

Genentech experience were the keys to getting the job. The positive interactions and chemistry with the senior partners at the bank also helped.

My Life as an Analyst

I did not wait for job offers that I hoped were forthcoming from other banks and immediately accepted this job. I surmised that the career prospects at a small bank might be better for someone just breaking into the finance world. A boutique investment bank is typically a small partnership with very focused research, investment banking, and stock trading operations. The role of a boutique bank in the mid-1990s was to be an initial public offering (IPO) comanager of choice. There was stiff competition from a number of great west coast banks, such as Montgomery, Robertson Stephens, and Hambrecht & Quist.

I was given a desk on the trading floor and a 1-day tutorial by the research associate who was leaving the firm, and then I was turned loose on the job. I was now expected to help the senior research analyst write research reports and to put together financial analyses to justify stock price targets for the stocks that we covered. I had no idea how complicated Excel spreadsheets could be, and I hadn't the slightest idea of how investment banks worked. I am glad that I am a quick learner because, only a few months after I started work, my boss, the senior research analyst, left the firm. Another associate and I were promoted to full-fledged research analysts. I had a real job on Wall Street!

I had to be at work before 5:00 A.M. because that was when our morning meeting started—before the New York stock markets opened at 9:30 A.M. eastern standard time. My day was never finished before 6:00 P.M. I routinely fell asleep in my soup. The work was amazingly great.

• • • • • • • • • • • • • • • • • • • •
"I routinely fell asleep in my soup."
• • • • • • • • • • • • • • • • • • • •

I learned that having a Ph.D. only got you so far with a sales force that had to sell your ideas to fund managers. You really had to understand what affected biotech stock price in a company on which you wrote research. After being laughed at a few times, I finally began to be taken seriously and that meant being taken around to fund managers to pitch ideas so that they would buy and sell stock through our trading floor. Pitching was all about "selling" my research and convincing fund managers and analysts to buy stocks that I had "buy" ratings on and to sell stocks that I had "hold" ratings on.

The other part of the job was trying to get biotech IPO business. This was 1997 and the tail end of an IPO market. The investment bankers and I flew around the country and met with a lot of companies that were hoping to raise money. We did get involved in a few deals and were paid a nice fee. The one IPO for which we were comanagers ultimately failed and filed for bankruptcy, which was a real learning experience about raising enough capital.

I learned that being a successful research analyst required an extrovert personality; a quick mind able to synthesize multiple influencing factors; the ability to write and create mathematical models to prove your point; and, not least, the ability to determine from very little information if the science, clinical data, and other fundamentals about a company were good. Companies sell hard since they covet research coverage, and sometimes it is not easy to see through to the facts. And I can't forget the importance of having the ability to generate large fees for the bank! The most rewarding thing about being a research analyst was getting it right.

• •

"The most rewarding thing about being a research analyst was getting it right."

• •

I made a few good calls on stocks and picked a few winners but had my share of bad calls. At about the time I finally felt like I knew what I was doing, the boutique investment bank was bought by a regional bank in Florida. I saw the writing on the wall and started looking for a new job. The Floridians had no idea what they had bought and had no idea how to run the business. This was the beginning of the end.

EVOLVING INTO A BANKER

After Genesis was purchased, I started putting out feelers for new job opportunities. I knew the research analysts at most of the investment banks, and I called them first. The research analyst at J.P. Morgan was interested in hiring someone to help cover some of the genomics stocks like Millennium Pharmaceuticals and Human Genome Sciences. Since I had covered a fair number of those stocks at Genesis, the analyst at JPM was quite keen on hiring me. I was introduced to the investment banker and capital markets person who covered biotech, and we really hit it off. A job offer was in the works when the research analyst left JPM. They quickly hired a replacement, a well-known research analyst who already had a team. So there went my research analyst position. However, the investment banker offered me a job in San Francisco with the investment banking team.

I had loved the investment banking aspects of my job at Genesis as well as the research, so I accepted the job. It turned out that my timing was perfect—Genesis laid everyone off shortly after I accepted the JPM job! My industry experience, my Ph.D., and my year covering biotech stocks all factored into me getting the JPM job. I knew a fair number of biotech management teams and knew a lot about the sector as a whole both from the science perspective and from the business perspective. The JPM health care group at the time had a big mergers and acquisitions (M&A) and public offering practice (and still does). So I was able to integrate into the team very quickly.

I got married 2 days after I started work at J.P. Morgan in 1998, right in the midst of an M&A transaction. I loved this job even more than the last one. JPM was a white shoe, old school, professionally run investment bank. And the biotech team (two investment bankers, a research analyst, and a capital markets person) was a small group that had recently come together and was part of the much larger, very successful health care team. It was also the middle of a major biotech financing down cycle, the perfect time to build a biotech practice from scratch.

"It was also the middle of a major biotech financing down cycle, the perfect time to build a biotech practice from scratch."

We pounded the pavement for months, and then everything came together at once. The M&A market took off as much as biotech M&A ever takes off. We were involved in a lot of transactions. And then Roche decided it could make a lot of money by a complicated buyback and spinout of Genentech. JPM was selected as the lead bank on the re-IPO of Genentech. That transaction has been credited with triggering the opening of the biggest biotech IPO market ever. It was a busy, crazy, wonderful time in the market, and the JPM team was the best team on the street. We had a lot of fun, worked together well as a team, and had a great book of business. The next 2 years were a real rollercoaster ride with one transaction after another, often overlapping.

DAILY TRANSACTIONS

On any given day, we were "pitching" M&A; valuing assets, drugs, or companies in an M&A transaction; pitching IPO business; drafting an S-1; or marketing or pricing a stock offering. Pitching M&A is all about coming up with interesting ideas for acquisitions. We would visit prospective clients with well thought through financial and strategic analyses of acquisition ideas. I typically spent half my time pitching or marketing M&A ideas and the other half executing transactions.

We were hired by companies to execute transactions once they had decided to pursue a particular acquisition idea or when they decided to sell the company. This involved a lot of financial modeling to come up with a fair price and to put together a viable strategy for the acquisition or sale.

Pitching IPO business was a completely different kettle of fish. There we were, selling not only the biotech team but the whole JPM machine. Many people are involved in IPOs. The bankers and analysts are only the front for a vast machine that not many people see. We, the bankers, were the main contact with the company that was thinking of going public. Our job was to get JPM hired by the company and then to help the company draft all the necessary documents required by the SEC, to help put together a "road show" presentation, and to accompany the management team on the road show. A lot of other people at JPM helped with all the other various processes that make up the complicated process of an IPO.

As the IPO window started to slam shut after Lexicon Genetics's billion dollar IPO that JPM led, and the market started to crash, we started to hear rumors that JPM was for sale. There had been rumors before, but nothing had ever happened. This time, as we were flying back to San Francisco from an IPO pitch, we found out that Chase Manhattan was indeed buying JPM.

FINALLY, VENTURE CAPITAL CALLS

Just before all that happened, the partners at Delphi Ventures called and asked me to interview with them. They were looking for a biotech partner. After a couple of meetings with them, I did not hear from them for a few months. We were having a really good year at JPM, so I did not think much of it. After the merger of JPM and Chase was finalized, Delphi called back to say that they were interested in discussing me joining them. This turned out to be a rather long, drawn-out decision. I had decided soon after leaving Genentech that venture capital was where I wanted to end up. Not knowing much about venture capital when I was at Genentech, it had seemed like the dream job. Venture capitalists seemed to be involved with many really interesting science projects, and they helped build nascent companies into big successful companies. This perception may have been naive, I know, but a lot of that has turned out to be true. However, I loved being an investment banker, and I had been promised a promotion at JPM.

> *"Venture capitalists seemed to be involved with many really interesting science projects, and they helped build nascent companies into big successful companies."*

There didn't seem to be much art to being an investment banker, but to be a really good one required a person to build really strong relationships with clients, be very analytical and innovative, and have the ability to market ideas and to execute them perfectly. The JPM organization was critical to the perfect execution. The Ph.D. after my name and the industry experience were an enormous help. The degree and background gave me credibility with biotech and pharmaceutical clients and gave me an edge over other investment bankers, particularly with M&A business. The Ph.D. title also gave me the ability to do diligence on prospective IPO clients.

Investment banking is supposed to be all about the next transaction. However, the most rewarding part of the job was the client relationships that transcended the job at JPM. I still get calls from clients to this day to tell me that they miss working with me and the JPM team. The biggest downside to being an investment banker was the arduous travel schedule. There were weeks when I spent every day on a plane going to a different place. My husband had taken to calling me his weekend wife.

The more time I spent with the Delphi partners made me realize that if venture capital was where I wanted to be, than this was the partnership to join. Delphi was one of the oldest focused health care funds in the country and has a great reputation. Further, every diligence call I made on Delphi was very positive. The partners at Delphi got rave reviews as board members and supportive venture investors; they were highly respected not only in the venture community but also in the biotech and medical device communities. I took a few months to decide, and I made a lot of diligence calls because joining a venture fund is more akin to getting married than simply accepting a new job. Partnerships last decades, and the financial ties are significant. Because I was offered a partner role at Delphi and the chance to help rebuild the biotech practice, my decision seemed to be made.

I joined Delphi Ventures in June 2001, 4 months pregnant. I had been nervous about telling the partners at Delphi about the baby since this development had happened between the time I interviewed for and was offered the job. As it turns out, the news was not a big deal because most of the partners at Delphi have families, and kids are a big part of people's lives at the organization. The 2½ years since then have been amazing, eventful, and all that I had hoped for. As much as I loved being a research analyst and an investment banker, I found that being a VC was what I had really wanted to be after all.

WHAT THE JOB IS LIKE

Being a VC allows me to use all the scientific training and all the skills I had learned in my previous jobs. Since Delphi is a small partnership, all the partners have their own scientific due diligence. So a science background is perfect for the job. Today, it is hard to get a job in venture capitalism without a Ph.D. or M.D. and some research experience. Finding companies to invest in is only the beginning. However, investment opportunities come in to Delphi from a lot of different places. People with whom Delphi partners have worked in the past are usually the ones who refer deals to us (the vast Delphi network!); however, other venture investors and contacts made through Delphi being known as a healthcare investment fund also refer deals to the company.

We look at a lot of deals every year and only invest in a few. These investments are in companies that meet stringent technological and scientific hurdles, that have great management teams, and that are very product oriented. We do a lot of scientific and clinical due diligence, as well as diligence on the people at the company. Our decision to invest in a company must be unanimous.

Once the partnership decides to invest in a company, the hard work begins. You typically get a seat on the board of directors if you are a large or lead investor. And as a director of the company, you are called on to help with numerous and varied decisions, including those on recruitment, strategic direction, financial priorities, clinical strategy, and other such topics. It is an enormous responsibility to be on a board, as well as a real team effort. I view the board as being part of the team that is integral to the success of a company. As a partner in a venture fund, you also are involved in raising new funds as each successive fund gets fully invested.

It is almost impossible to describe a typical day in the life of a VC, which is why it is so enjoyable. Every day brings new challenges and opportunities. You see cutting-edge science as it happens, spend time with extremely smart entrepreneurs, and truly help build something that will have a major impact on millions of lives. We typically co-invest with other venture capital funds and have worked with almost every fund in the country that invests in health care. So nurturing relationships with partners in other venture funds is important.

So, I have found my dream job, helping in a very small way to build a piece of the biotech sector. Unfortunately, I won't know how successful I am going to be at it for another 5 years, at least: the measure of a VC's success is in how much money your fund returns to the investors in the fund, which is a measure of the success of the companies in which you have invested. Biotech companies typically stay private for 4 to 7 years before they can go public in an IPO, which is when venture investors can sell the stock. If biotech cycles stay true to form, then investments I have made in the last 2½ years will come public, and we will be able to distribute stock to investors in Delphi Ventures in a few years.

7

· · · · · · · · · ·

INVESTMENT BANKING:

Dreams and Reality

· · · · · · · · · · · · · · · ·

Peter Drake, Ph.D.[*]

Executive Vice President; Former Managing Director and President,
Vector Securities (ret.)

I have always loved science. As an adolescent, I enjoyed learning about aquatic biology and botany fishing in the solitary streams of southern Missouri. But the real fun began as a teenager when I got a summer job in 1967 as a complete grunt in the Surgical Research Laboratory at St. John's Mercy Medical Center in suburban St. Louis. I was 14 years old and had a job where I could wear that all-important white laboratory coat.

That coat was the only ego-boosting aspect of that first job, which tested my resolve to become a research assistant. Much of the experimental work in the lab involved surgical procedures on dogs, which meant I was assigned to the beagle patrol. Yes, I cleaned the dog pens daily in the sweltering heat of the St. Louis summer. I passed this first test, and the following summer I was rewarded with the air conditioning of the lab and the minimum wage ($2.50/hour).

After learning the rudiments of chemistry, biology, and physics in high school, in 1972 I headed off to Bowdoin College in Brunswick, Maine, intending to major in biology and later attend medical school. I was determined to choose a career path distinct from my father, who, as a farm boy with only a high school education, was one of the founding employees of

[*]Updated for second edition by Cynthia Robbins-Roth

McDonnell Aircraft Corporation, known today as McDonnell Douglas (or, since the recent merger, Boeing).

But my dream of attending medical school was dealt a severe blow in my first semester of freshman year. Despite working harder than I ever had, my grades were straight Cs. I still loved science, but it seemed clear that my academic interests had to be applied to a career that didn't require the straight-A record needed to get into medical school. I changed to focus on the pursuit of science as an intellectual passion, all the while keeping an eye toward other career applications open to an undergraduate double major in Biology and Russian.

> *"I still loved science, but it seemed clear that my academic interests had to be applied to a career that did not require the straight-A record needed to get into medical school."*

THE PLAN

By my senior year in 1976, it was clear that two areas of science—molecular biology and neuroscience—were poised to undergo a revolution. It was also clear to me that these scientific advances would lead to remarkable opportunities in industry. So my plan was to get a Ph.D. and position myself to capture new career opportunities in the industrial applications of biological sciences.

I chose to attend graduate school at Bryn Mawr College (with an all-female undergraduate school) in the fall of 1976 for two reasons: first, I could pursue a double degree in biochemistry and neurobiology with professors I truly admired, and, second, after 8 years at an all-male prep school and 4 years at Bowdoin (where mine was the second class to admit women), I could instantly improve my odds of getting a date.

I spent my first 2 years in the advanced seminar program, which had a strong emphasis on independent study. My summers were spent at the Marine Biological Laboratory (MBL) in Woods Hole, Massachusetts, working on experiments to support my Ph.D. thesis.

It was in Woods Hole in the summer of 1978, while sitting on the beach reading the Sunday *New York Times*, that I learned about the first sign of a convergence of biology and industry. A patent covering an oil-eating bacteria had been granted to General Electric. This so-called Chakabarty patent was the first granted on a new life form. It was absolutely clear to me that if one could patent new biological discoveries, industrial applications were not far behind.

THE MENTORS

The harsh reality in 1980 was that I had a Ph.D., a fiancée, and a job in the Department of Anatomy and Developmental Biology at Case Western Reserve Medical School paying $13,380. By accepting this job, I allowed my career to move along a classic academic route in pursuit of my love for science. Unfortunately, I had achieved the "easy" part of my plan—the advanced degree—but I lacked the career-specific vision and the means to execute this vision.

I didn't know it at the time, but what I needed was a mentor. Within the span of a few months, I found two mentors. The first would provide me with the business vision to pursue my goal, and the second would give me the intellectual confidence to execute the plan. My business mentor took me back to St. Louis. Dr. Louis Fernandez was named chairman of the board of Monsanto in 1980, capping a distinguished career at the company where he began as a bench scientist. Monsanto was positioning itself for the future of agricultural biotechnology under Dr. Fernandez's leadership. He was also on the board of directors of Biogen, at the time a fledgling biotechnology start-up in Cambridge, Massachusetts, led by the Nobel Prize laureate, Dr. Walter Gilbert.

In high school, I had often played tennis with Dr. Fernandez. So I took a risk and wrote him a letter describing my interest in combining a background in science with work in industry. About 5 days later, I received a return letter inviting me to a meeting in St. Louis. During our 2-hour discussion, we spoke about the coming revolution in the biotechnology industry and Monsanto's keen interest in capitalizing on the opportunity.

Dr. Fernandez told me to pursue my post-doc, but also to take concurrently some accounting and finance courses. He told me that Monsanto would have many opportunities for someone with my skill set, but if he were in my shoes, he would go to Wall Street and become an investment analyst. His view was that the biotechnology industry was going to emerge as an important new industry with significant capital requirements. Also, there were going to be many public biotechnology companies in need of analytical and scientific insight. Well there it was, presented on a silver platter—undeniably the best advice that I have ever received. I now had an executable plan.

• •
"Dr. Fernandez told me to pursue my post-doc, but also to take concurrently some accounting and finance courses."
• •

My other mentor's influence was gradual in developing, but his teaching had a profound impact on the skills I draw upon as an analyst and investor. Dr. Raymond Lasek, a noted neuroscientist, taught me to work and think independently; to be curious and creative; to write succinctly and to communicate clearly with strong and persuasive selling skills; to take risks and to be scared; and above all, to challenge the wisdom of the status quo.

THE FIRST BREAK

During the 3 years I spent in Dr. Lasek's lab, I learned completely new fields of science, but most important, I learned that I could teach myself almost anything. My research project was highly interdisciplinary, focusing on neuroscience, cell biology, and biochemistry. At night and on weekends, I followed the stock market, invested in health care stocks, and studied the ascent of the biotechnology industry.

I prepared a résumé, spent months refining my cover letter (the written description of what I wanted to do in a career), and interviewed for a variety of industrial and consulting positions. This was all intended as preparation for the trip to Wall Street. I learned about the Wall Street firms covering health care and biotechnology stocks; I studied the backgrounds of the biotechnology analysts; I talked to investment professionals to learn about the investment process.

From this effort, I knew that I had a deficiency, and curiously enough it was an academic deficiency. My scholastic background lacked an academic pedigree recognizable on Wall Street. Specifically, I had not attended an Ivy League school or a leading business school. Either or both of these represented an entrance ticket to a job on the Street. Further, my family lacked Wall Street contacts. But an MBA seemed out of reach—I was 29, married for 3 years, and still making less than $15,000. I was, however, hungry and resourceful.

I then learned about a summer program sponsored by the Wharton Business School at the University of Pennsylvania, designed to train those with Ph.D.s in business fundamentals. Instinctively, I knew the potential importance of this program. My summer in Philadelphia at Wharton was fantastic—tremendous teachers, dedicated administrators, and a diverse and an enthusiastic group of colleagues. The time was right to put this all to work.

I interviewed with three Wall Street firms, and I chose to join a distinguished research department at Kidder, Peabody, & Company as a biotechnology analyst. My group leader and Wall Street mentor, Arnie Snider, later told me that my cover letter and résumé stood out among the many people Kidder was interviewing. The refinement of these two documents over the previous year had paid off! In addition, I interviewed well, I was knowledgeable about the securities business and the other Wall Street firms, and I had a view of biotech stocks and an understanding of the biotech industry.

After I was hired, George Boyd, my boss, showed me my office, gave me free reign in defining the stocks I would follow, and left me alone for a year as I traveled throughout the United States visiting companies and attending scientific meetings. I made $85,000 my first year in the business. I was hooked!

THE SKILL SET REQUIRED BY AN ANALYST

Having hired and trained scores of analysts over the past 15 years, I would say that there is no single trait or skill set necessary for success. In fact, I will admit that having been the oldest biotech analyst on Wall Street does not mean that I have all the answers or that the learning process is over.

Before describing the various important characteristics of being an effective analyst, I will start with the critically important things I have learned. Arnie Snider taught me that there is a difference between companies and stocks. Biotech companies are about people, technology platforms, business and financial strategies, and products; stocks are pieces of paper. An analyst's primary job is to recommend stocks that go up in value and to avoid stocks that go down in value.

It is also critical to recognize that in the investment business, we live in a relative world as opposed to an absolute world. By this, I mean that institutional investors are supremely performance–oriented, and they are graded on the basis of the performance of their funds relative to the market's overall performance. If an analyst's recommendation is up 25% when the S&P 500 has appreciated 30%, that means the stock has underperformed the market. I taught our analysts and investment bankers that we are actually in the paper business—we analyze it, we trade it, and we issue it. Consultants analyze companies and strategies, but securities analysts are stock pickers.

The next step in the process is communication—both verbal and written. When an analyst has found a stock that he or she believes is undervalued (the stock price does not reflect the company's value), the key is to market the idea to both the firm's salespeople and directly to institutional clients. If an investment idea can't be packaged and communicated succinctly, the idea will not rise above the competitive noise level of other analysts at other investment firms pitching their ideas.

Beyond these big-picture issues, the skill set for a biotech analyst includes being honest and professional, having a strong work ethic, maintaining a competitive spirit, being inquisitive and skeptical, having a solid accounting and finance background (i.e., an MBA.), having a strong knowledge of science and technology, paying attention to detail, and having strong financial modeling skills.

A TYPICAL DAY AS AN ANALYST

The brokerage business begins with the morning research meeting. Analysts stand in front of the salespeople and traders and make a 2- to 5-minute sales pitch focusing on the reasons to buy or sell a particular stock. Then, salespeople and analysts hit the phones, marketing the idea to institutional clients on the "buy-side"—specifically, portfolio managers and analysts.

Nearly every day, analysts speak with companies, either in phone conferences with the top management contacts or in one-on-one meetings with these executives in the office or during site visits at company headquarters. These contacts with company managements become the source of future comments for the morning meeting. News items by companies that emerge during the day are analyzed, and comments to the sales force are directed to institutional clients. Finally, considerable time is spent in writing formal research reports.

A typical day spent out of the office involves one of three activities: site visits at companies to meet with key senior management officials; attending industry conferences and/or scientific meetings; and marketing to institutional clients in group meetings (e.g., at breakfast, lunch, and/or dinner) or in one-on-one meetings. Herein lies, in my opinion, the most enjoyable (and potentially the most stressful) part of the job.

Marketing trips are known for their hectic pace. A typical west coast trip would begin with a later afternoon flight to San Diego and a dinner meeting with 10 to 12 clients. A 4:00 A.M. wake-up call allows for a review of the content for the morning research call at 5:00 A.M. After three one-to-one hour-long meetings with separate clients, the salesman would then drive to Los Angeles for three additional separate meetings. Finally, a dinner meeting would end the day at around 9:00 P.M. The next day, an early flight to Portland, Oregon, would allow for several private meetings, a group lunch, and then a flight to Seattle for a dinner meeting. Four separate meetings the following morning lead to a flight to Denver for a full day (i.e., six to eight one-on-one meetings), and we would then fly back on a late-night flight to Chicago. Many of these meetings might be contentious (depending on the state of the stock market at the time), so an analyst must possess both a thick skin and endurance.

From the financial reward perspective, it is common for industry-specific analysts (e.g., biotech, medical devices, health care services, and so forth) to start with a combination salary/bonus of $150,000 to $200,000; some of the big banks pay less (prestige factor). From there, it is a matter of how much revenue you generate for the firm. In one way or another, analysts and bankers are rewarded based on the money they bring into the firm, which can mean some pretty big bucks. A good stock picker has the opportunity to double or triple his or her initial salary, based on time at the firm and performance; bonuses can get as high as $2 million/year if you generate a lot of business.

WHERE I HOPE TO GO FROM HERE

I joined Kidder, Peabody, & Company in October 1983; I loved the firm, and I made lasting friendships with colleagues and clients. I was honored by becoming a partner within 2 years and achieving the number 1 ranking on the Institutional Investor All-Star Team.

I cofounded Vector Securities International, Inc., in 1988 with two remarkable partners, colleagues, and friends—Ted Berghorst, an investment banker, and Jim Foght, Ph.D., a former pharmaceutical executive turned investment banker. Together, we have formed the Later Stage Equity Funds I and II with a total of $230 million under management, designed for private negotiated investments in life sciences companies. In addition, we cofounded Deerfield Partners, a $2 billion company on health care hedge fund run by Arnie Snider in New York City. Vector Securities International has been involved in more than 300 transactions and has raised roughly $5 billion in capital for the life sciences industry.

I spent the first 6 years being an analyst and running the research department as director of research. This worked as long as Vector was a small organization. As the company grew, the research department expanded to 20 professionals. I had to decide if I wanted to oversee the management of the research department or go back full-time as an analyst. By the end of 1994, I chose to be an analyst, and we hired the person who had run research at Drexel and was CEO of County NatWest Securities.

My responsibilities as executive vice president and biotech analyst included participating on the operating committee and the board of directors. The operating committee met weekly for a couple of hours to oversee and review the firm's operations. I was also a partner in the Later-Stage Equity Fund. We closed the second fund in this family with $130 million and Genentech as the lead special partner. I had followed Genentech for years as an analyst; I no longer cover the organization as an analyst, but it was showing its faith in Vector by investing a substantial amount. We spent the last quarter of 1993, all of 1994, and part of 1995 raising $51 million for Fund I, providing investors with a performance that is up 90%. This paid off—it took us only 4 months to raise $180 million for Fund II.

In 1998 and 1999, a wave of consolidation swept through the investment banking industry, and Vector also participated in this trend. We had struggled to build our trading operations to compete with the large, well-capitalized firms on Wall Street. Accordingly, in mid-1999, we consummated a deal with Prudential Securities; we became a "firm within a firm," called Prudential Vector Healthcare, and in 2000 quadrupled our revenue from our old base at Vector. The firm was thriving, and our competitive position was greatly enhanced. However, by year-end 2000, Prudential decided to exit the investment banking business. Because a component of our merger deal involved an up-front payment and an earn out from the profits of Prudential Vector Healthcare, we were able to negotiate a "buy-out of our earn-out." My banking partners left Prudential, and I remained with my colleagues in the research department as a managing director and biotech analyst. Because I loved the research process and the "Wall Street game," I stayed at Prudential throughout 2001 and retired in early 2002.

Today, I am in the "give back" phase of my career. I sit on several boards of directors of private and public healthcare companies and act as an "angel" investor helping to finance and guide small companies as they grow. I remain an optimist at heart but recognize the extreme challenges necessary to build a stand-alone biotech company. The rules regarding Wall Street and research have changed dramatically in the wake of Elliott Spitzer's negotiated settlement with the brokerage industry, but the name of the game will never change—do independent research on industry trends and specific companies, translate this knowledge into money-making ideas for clients, and try to have fun.

Chapter

8

· · · · · · · · · ·

HOW I BECAME AN ANALYST:

Science-Based Investment Advising

· · · · · · · · · · · · · · · · ·

Mary Ann Gray, Ph.D.
Gray Strategic Advisors, LLC
Former Biotechnology Analyst, SBC Warburg Dillon Read, Inc.

THE EARLY YEARS

Even as a child, I was interested in how things work. When I was 6, my father got an electric razor for Christmas. That afternoon, my parents found me in my room with pieces of the razor scattered around. When asked what on Earth I thought I was doing, I replied, "I just wanted to see how it worked." Over time, my interests evolved into discovering how the human body works. Living in South Carolina from age 11 through college, I was never really exposed to scientists. Consequently, I thought that the only way to delve into the mysteries of the body was to become a physician. Since I was very shy, the thought of dealing with strangers was not appealing, and I became attracted to pathology (dead people are a lot less threatening!). I settled on becoming a pathologist as early as the seventh grade.

High school was not a wonderful experience for me, and I decided to leave high school after my junior year and enter the University of South Carolina as a non-high school graduate in the summer of 1969. Of course, my major was biology.

After my freshman year, I got married and had a child at age 18. Needless to say, this caused some changes in my plans to attend medical school and become a research pathologist. After my son was born, I returned to school right away but had to attend at night so that my mother could babysit while my husband worked evenings. Back then, science courses were not offered at night, so I worked on my electives for about a year and a half. When my son was 2, I went back to school full-time, and I graduated in December 1973.

BEGINNING A CAREER

Medical school seemed out of the question at that point, so I did the next best thing—I became a medical technologist at Moncreif Army Hospital in Fort Jackson, South Carolina. This allowed me to become familiar with the general workings of a laboratory as I rotated through the various departments. I also got to deal with patients when it was my turn to go on the floors and draw the early morning blood samples. More importantly, I got to work with pathologists. When there was an autopsy to do, most of the technologists became very busy with other things. I, however, was always eager to help. Our pathologist was a wonderful teacher, and I learned a great deal about anatomy and pathology during these sessions in the morgue.

I soon became bored with the routine of the hospital laboratory and tried to find a job doing "real" research. I moved to Northern Virginia to be near the National Cancer Institute (NCI), and I started working for a contract research firm. Our specific task was to manage the preclinical toxicology of new anticancer drugs being developed by NCI. We did not perform the tests ourselves but selected various subcontracting labs, and then we provided an independent assessment of the results, including hematology clinical chemistry and pathology reports.

"I soon became bored with the routine of the hospital laboratory and tried to find a job doing 'real' research."

This job was one of the many turning points in my career. I was given as much responsibility as I could handle, and my boss, an excellent toxicologist, supported me. I also worked hand-in-hand with scientists at the NCI and at various pharmaceutical companies and universities. It was with the help of these wonderful friends and mentors that I gained the courage to go back to school 7 years after receiving my bachelor's degree.

Since I was a little uneasy about returning to school, I chose to attend the University of Vermont. At that time, Vermont had the characteristics that I was looking for in a graduate program, and two of my former colleagues were on the faculty. The pharmacology department was small, but

Vermont had an excellent regional cancer center, and the laboratory and clinical staff interacted a great deal. I felt that I would be able to learn how to gear my research toward applications that would be important in patient treatment. I was not interested in true basic research, but in transplanting the principles discovered by the basic scientists into patient care.

My graduate school project evolved from my previous work with the anticancer drug doxorubicin and its analogues in an attempt to find a drug with reduced cardiotoxicity. My focus was the potential mechanism of this cardiotoxicity and ways to reduce it, and I developed models to screen new compounds for improved characteristics. I continued to pursue this research during a year of post-doctoral research at Northwestern University Medical School, and then I expanded this work to working on other anticancer agents with Dr. Alan Sartorelli at Yale University School of Medicine. I had never aspired to an academic career, and after 2 more years as a post-doc, I decided that it was time to make my break into the corporate world.

THE BUSINESS OF SCIENCE

Because of my experience with antitumor drugs and my expertise in developing animal models, I was hired by a private biotechnology company to preside over the preclinical development of certain monoclonal antibody conjugates.

The biotechnology world was fascinating in a number of respects. The work was focused, and the goals were clear. The company had approximately 70 employees when I joined, and the atmosphere was very collegial. We were all pulling together toward the same end, getting a product on the market. Project management meetings exposed us to input from all areas of the company. I worked with clinicians to design animal models that would be better predicators of results in

"Wearing many hats in a small organization is a wonderful way to gain at least some appreciation of all aspects of building a business."

humans, I learned what things were important to our fledgling marketing and sales group, and I learned how to manage both a budget and people. Wearing many hats in a small organization is a wonderful way to gain at least some appreciation of all aspects of building a business.

During my time at the biotechnology company, management decided to pursue an initial public offering (IPO). This was a fascinating experience for me because my involvement with Wall Street until that time was limited to brief scans of the business pages in the local newspaper. It became even more interesting when we tried to close the deal in October 1987, the day of the big stock market crash. Not surprisingly, the deal was postponed until a better time.

After a few years, the fortunes of the biotech industry and this company in particular diminished. The products took longer to develop and were more expensive than expected. We went through one downsizing that was extremely painful, especially in a small company where all of the employees knew each other fairly well. Even worse, the first cut did not achieve the goals, and there was a second layoff only a few months later. The morale of the remaining employees was at an all-time low. I decided that it was time for me to move on.

In considering my options, I was looking for something new. I had done the academic thing as well as contract research and I'd worked for a hospital laboratory and a biotech company. What was missing? Aha! Working for a major pharmaceutical company was something I had not yet tried. That decision led to a move to Schering-Plough in the relatively new tumor biology department, where I was in charge of the preclinical work on potential new treatments for cancer. Most people make a move from the pharmaceutical industry to the biotechnology industry, not the other way around—and now I know why. At a smaller company, everyone tends to work together. People wear many hats, and you are expected to voice your opinions to help keep projects on track. It is a simple matter to talk to the vice president of research or even the CEO whenever you wish to express an opinion.

In a large pharmaceutical corporation, however, the organizational and team approaches do not usually kick in until lead compounds are selected and handed over to the clinical development group. Research is much less directed, and I felt as though I were spinning my wheels. I felt that I was moving farther away than ever from my goal of developing products to treat patients.

THE RIGHT PLACE AT THE RIGHT TIME

As I was trying to decide what my next move would be, I talked to a friend who had recently attended a meeting where several Wall Street biotechnology analysts had given presentations. She told me that it sounded like the ideal job for me—they get to work on a variety of projects (hence no boredom), they travel (I like to travel), and they get to interact with a diverse and interesting group of people (I have definitely outgrown my shyness).

It sounded interesting, so I begin to write letters to the analysts asking for information. Most important for me was whether they thought it necessary that I obtain an M.B.A. before I could move into an analyst slot. Having spent a good portion of my life in school and having just finished paying for my son's college, I was not anxious to tackle another 2 years of school and, more importantly, to lose income.

I received several polite replies, but in December 1991, I received a call from the analyst at Kidder, Peabody, & Company. This analyst had a Ph.D. *and* an M.B.A. At this time, the biotechnology market was really "hot," and investment banks were working on numerous biotech IPOs. Evaluating all of the existing and potential companies was too much for one person, and Kidder, Peabody, & Company needed help. Again, I asked about the need for an M.B.A. and was assured that the scientific expertise was more important at this point. (I have also come to realize that my experience working in the both the biotechnology and pharmaceutical industries is equally important.) In February 1992, I left Schering-Plough for Wall Street.

During my first few months, I was meeting with companies and evaluating technology nonstop. However, things quickly came to a standstill when numerous clinical disasters caused the industry to fall out of favor with investors. On the positive side, this lull gave me an opportunity to get my feet wet without too much intense pressure. It was a good thing I got this time to come up the learning curve, since 6 months later the senior analyst left, and I was on my own.

After about 3 years, a change was forced upon me. In late 1994, Paine Webber, another investment bank, bought Kidder, Peabody, & Company and brought in its own biotech analyst—suddenly, I was out of a job. While in the past I have always been ready to move on after about 3 years, this time I was not even close to getting bored. Had I finally found the right job? And how could I stay in the game despite the merger?

Because being an analyst is a little like being an independent operator, I decided to see if I could use my experience and contacts to run a consulting service. I formed Biologic, Inc., and began to work on a broad range of projects for numerous clients. These projects included developing investor relations strategies, writing private placement documents, providing valuations for potential acquisitions, and writing a newsletter.

After a successful first year, I was getting to the point where I needed to hire a full-time assistant. I had never before been responsible for paying someone else's salary, and it made me a little nervous. As I was wrestling with this decision, I received a call from a former Kidder colleague, now at Dillon Read. (The majority of Kidder's health care team ended up at Dillon Read.) Would I like to come back to Wall Street? I must say, the answer would probably have been "No" if it had been anyone else asking. But with this group, I knew what I was getting into, and I knew that it would work as it had in the past. I have now been at Dillon Read a little over a year, and I have just learned that SBC Warburg is buying the company. (See, I do not have to keep changing jobs now; my job keeps changing on its own!)

WHAT DOES A BIOTECHNOLOGY ANALYST DO?

In general, the job of a biotechnology analyst is to evaluate biotechnology for investors. The bottom line is whether an investor can make money by investing in a particular company. The trick is to figure out which of the many companies represent the best investing opportunity—and it is not always just a question of which company has the best science.

Many people think that we have armies of analysts for each industry, but this is not true. Most firms now have two analysts who may be supported by one or two research associates. With more than 350 publicly traded biotechnology companies for investors to choose from, the task of selecting the best investment opportunities with limited resources can be daunting.

I think of my job as having three major parts: research, marketing, and corporate finance. At various points, the time spent on each part can vary a great deal. One common thread is that there is never enough time. In this fast-paced business, you always feel that something is being neglected.

Research involves a number of activities, including company-specific research and industry research. When evaluating a company, you must look at the products it is developing, the technology that it uses, its management team, and its business strategy. The first source of information is usually the company, but facts need to be verified by independent sources.

Researching a company is the area that is most closely related to scientific research, where scientific skills are readily useful. The type of information that you are evaluating may be in the form of scientific publications, abstracts, or company presentations. Keep in mind that the goal here is to eventually make money for investors, so no matter how scientifically elegant a project may be, you will have trouble ahead if the ultimate product is not clinically useful, is too costly, or is otherwise unsuitable for use in a patient population that is large enough. It is also important to have a broad scientific background. The technology you are evaluating will not always be in your area of expertise. I was trained as a pharmacologist according to classical principles, and this broad background has been useful in evaluating information from areas outside the cancer field, such as neuroscience, virology, and the like.

•••••••••••••••••••••
"It is also important to have a broad scientific background. The technology you are evaluating will not always be in your area of expertise."
•••••••••••••••••••••

There is never enough time to evaluate these areas, and you can't possibly do enough reading to quickly become an expert in an entirely new field. Therefore, it is important to develop good instincts and a strong network of scientific and medical colleagues on whom you can depend.

I also try to attend several scientific and medical meetings each year. The medical meetings tend to be more useful because I can get a feel for the state of the art in the treatment of various diseases and what technology physicians are excited about. These meetings also give me a chance to speak with experts in various fields about technology that I am evaluating. When data from one of the companies that I follow are presented, I am always very interested in the questions asked by the experts in the audience.

In addition to evaluating the scientific feasibility of a company's products, you must also evaluate the market potential with these possible questions:

- How many patients have the disease?
- How are they treated now?
- Will the new product be useful for all patients or only for a small subset?
- Is the new product better than existing therapy?
- Will doctors use the product?
- How much will the product cost?
- Will insurance companies and HMOs pay for the product?

These are questions that most scientists are not used to asking, but they are crucial to evaluating a new product. It is important to think practically and to understand how physicians treat patients.

Decision to Invest

Okay, assume that the company has a potentially great product that looks like it is going to work, physicians think the product will be useful, and the product saves money so it will be reimbursed. Does management have a plan to get the product into the marketplace and the experience to execute that plan?

This is one of the more subjective parts of the job, but it is also very important. The managers of a biotech company have to play many roles, and they must communicate with a diverse audience. I try to rely on track records as much as possible, and I follow a company's progress for a while before making a "buy/don't buy" decision. This requires numerous meetings with management to define their goals, which entails following up on progress over time. Are they overly optimistic about timelines and costs? Is there always an excuse for not achieving milestones? Or do they always meet their stated goals on or ahead of schedule? I must also admit that gut feelings play a role, but it is crucial to develop a trust in management.

Okay, now assume that the company has products in the pipeline, and they have put together a great team. Now we need to look at whether investors funding this enterprise actually make money. For most biotechnology companies (with only about six exceptions), profits will be made in the future. Trying to project future earnings, much less to determine their value today, is a difficult task that involves some fortune-telling skills. Public companies rely on investments from the public to bring their products to market. This is a costly enterprise that requires $250 million to $450 million and usually requires 10 to 12 years for just one product. What is the company's plan for financing this development process? How will management balance investment in research and development of new products with making a profit for investors as soon as is feasible?

After all of this analysis has taken place and you have decided that the company is a winner, you must explain how you arrived at that conclusion to a diverse audience composed of some very naïve laypeople, some very sophisticated institutional investors, and everyone in between. You must write a report that conveys the important points without losing the attention of people who don't have time to read through your pithy prose. You must tell the story of what the company does clearly, and you must also explain why you feel that it is the right time to invest. Investors need to know what likely events will increase the value of the company and the stock price over the next 6 to 12 months. (This is a long time to an investor.)

The companies that you "cover" include those for which you are actively writing reports and notes to investors, those for which you have a detailed financial model, and those for which you have made an investment recommendation. This recommendation is usually to buy, sell, hold, or a variation thereof depending on your firm (different firms may use different terminology to avoid saying "sell"). A single analyst typically can cover from 10 to 15 companies on a regular basis, depending on the amount of support that he or she has.

Marketing Stocks to Buyers

All of this research leads into the second major aspect of the sell-side analyst job, which is to market these stocks to buyers. (Buy-side analysts work directly with portfolio managers and institutional investors to decide which stocks to buy.) Once you have these great investment ideas, you must communicate this enthusiasm to the investors so that they will buy (or sell) the stock.

The first line of communication is your firm's institutional sales force. These people have specific client institutions with which they are in daily contact concerning buy, sell, and hold advice across all sectors. Your ideas are transferred to the sales force via your written reports, morning notes (brief comments on the impact of specific news events on stocks), or other specific comments—a change in earnings estimates or something that has changed your opinion of the stock-on companies that you officially cover.

In addition to the written reports and notes, you must also talk to your sales force. This takes place at a daily meeting at approximately 7:30 A.M. east coast time (4:30 A.M. for west coast analysts calling in)—hence the term "the morning call." The meeting takes place early so that the information that is relayed by the analysts becomes the subject of the sales force's daily calls to their institutional accounts. This information must be relayed to the clients before the stock market opens at 9:30 A.M. (6:30 on the west coast) to allow clients to take action immediately. In addition to having the salesperson call the clients with news, it is also important for the analyst to call certain key clients directly. It is important for an institutional investor to get to know and trust the analyst who is providing the information on which the investor may risk a great deal of money.

Research on general trends in the industry is also important, and you should consider the following questions:

- What are the current areas of interest (or disinterest) for investors?
- What kinds of companies are paying off now?
- What characteristics do successful companies have in common?
- How do investors define the profile of the ideal company? (This changes frequently, depending on how well past investments are doing.)
- Is biotech a worthwhile investment?
- How do you choose the right companies in which to invest?

Written reports on industry trends and fundamentals are helpful for investors, but they also help you to formulate and articulate clear, concise opinions about your industry.

In addition to written reports, morning notes, and discussions with the sales force and clients, it is important to visit certain clients on a regular basis. Face-to-face meetings help build the relationship and generate trust. Clients can also be a valuable source of information. A typical marketing meeting can be a valuable two-way exchange of information.

Corporate Financing

Corporate finance is the third portion of the job. The corporate finance group, also called bankers, helps client companies raise money, advises them on mergers and acquisitions, and provides crucial strategic advice. Depending on the firm, the analyst may or may not be heavily involved in certain corporate finance decisions.

Initial public offerings tend to require the most work. I like to meet with, and get to know, interesting private companies early. This allows me the time to make some judgments about management and to follow the company's progress even before the company becomes a banking client. It also gives the bankers and me a chance to guide the company through the process of deciding on the right time to approach the public markets and to decide what their other alternatives might be.

Once a decision has been made to go forward with a public offering, I tend to participate heavily in .the "due diligence" process. This involves numerous conference calls with collaborators, scientific founders, corporate partners, physicians, and others to evaluate the company. This process is somewhat akin to checking references. I also go through all of my typical research steps, including building a detailed financial model of the company.

After due diligence is completed, the company must write a prospectus, a document filed with the Securities and Exchange Commission (SEC) that is given to potential investors. The business section of this document describes the company in detail, and it is important that this section be clear and understandable. I like to take part at least in the initial stages of drafting this document. The next step is to prepare a 30-minute slide presentation that will be used to describe the company to potential investors around the world in a grueling ordeal called a "road show."

During the road show, the company will give this presentation numerous times in several key cities throughout the United States and Europe. Some of the presentations will be given to groups of investors during breakfast or lunch. Other presentations will be one-on-one meetings with key investors. I like to have some input in the slide show, but I do not typically go on the road show. I do make follow-up calls to investors who meet with the company so that I can answer any questions and describe why I feel that the company is a good investment. Once the offering is completed, this company is added to my coverage list, and I write a detailed research report.

Other activities related to corporate finance include follow-on offering for existing public companies and evaluating potential merger or acquisition candidates for our clients.

POSITIVES AND NEGATIVES

As you can tell, there is never enough time to do everything as thoroughly as you would like. This keeps the job exciting, but it is sometimes frustrating, especially if you are a scientist who is used to examining every last detail. The ability to disseminate information rapidly is important and has to be balanced with a well-thought-out opinion.

The job requires working long hours. The morning call is at 7:30 A.M., and if you didn't write a morning note on a topic the night before, you have to come in early enough to have it written and approved prior to the call. The evenings are often a time to catch up on reading after the phones have stopped ringing, and frequently there is a dinner meeting with the managers of a company that lasts until 9:00 or 10:00 P.M. In addition, visiting companies, attending scientific and medical meetings, visiting clients, and attending and presenting at industry conferences require a great deal of travel.

The job requires dedication because of the hours and amount of energy spent to keep on top of rapid advances and competition. On the positive side, it is never boring. If you grow tired of working on a medical topic, you can focus on a financial model, or you can call a client to chat about the industry.

> *"The job requires dedication because of the hours and amount of energy spent to keep on top of rapid advances and competition."*

Job security is nonexistent. Every time the biotech sector tanks, many banks shed their biotech analysts. They rehire when the sector heats up again, but this is not much consolation. Also, as I experienced, the merger mania in the banking world can throw a monkey wrench into your career plans.

How much are analysts paid? This is a tough question to answer because pay can vary greatly and rumors abound. In general, analysts receive a base salary plus a bonus. The base salaries range from about $30,000 to $60,000 for a research associate, $60,000 to $90,000 for a junior analyst, and $90,000 to $125,000 and more for a senior analyst. The base salary is similar to that for most other types of jobs, and there is a range for each level. The names of the levels vary among firms, but typically the grades include research associate, associate analyst, vice president, senior vice president, and managing director.

The bonus is the more difficult part to figure out. It depends on many factors, and most firms do not have a preset formula for determining the bonus level. In addition, different portions of the job can be more or less important at different firms. The bonus pool—the amount of money the firm dedicates to bonuses—is influenced by how profitable the firm has been that year, so bonuses can vary greatly from year to year.

The size of an individual analyst's bonus depends on things you can't control, such as how well the investment banking business in the sector is doing that year. Investment banks make a lot of money by taking companies public and conducting follow-on offerings, so analysts who work on several offerings usually get a small piece of each fee as a part of their bonus. Some firms emphasize the rankings published in *Institutional Investor,* a publication that annually picks the top three analysts in each sector according to votes from institutional investors. Some see this as a popularity contest, but it is designed to pick those analysts who help institutional investors make wise investment choices.

Other factors that determine the bonus include quantity and quality of reports published, the opinion of the sales force on how helpful the analyst is to them, and the performance of the analyst's recommendations regarding their covered companies.

Bonuses vary from about $50,000 to $1 million for senior analysts, but in general, they are at least several hundred thousand dollars. This makes an average analyst's compensation in the range of $300,000 to $500,000, but there are always many exceptions.

However, there are some who believe that good analysts are paid whatever amount it takes to get them to stay with the firm. This creates an atmosphere much like professional sports, where analysts often jump ship to a higher bidder. Rumors of $1 million signing bonuses and multimillion dollar contracts abound.

Writing is important. You must be able to write in a style that is easily understood and that conveys the gist of very complex issues in a way that holds the readers' interest. You also must write quickly, for time is, in fact, money in this business.

Biotechnology is a diverse industry, both in the technologies involved and the people. We can all appreciate the differences between a scientist who is happy in the lab with no one to bother him or her and a CEO who has the gift of gab. As an analyst, it is important to be able to walk in many different worlds and to communicate in different languages. It is the combination of these different worlds in the biotechnology industry that I find fascinating.

As scientists, we are taught to question, and that is also a key attribute for an analyst. Even when you listen to presentations outside of your field of expertise, your scientific training should allow you to evaluate the information that is presented and ask the right questions. In addition to my scientific training, my work in both the biotechnology and pharmaceutical industries has provided me with the experience necessary to ask the right questions regarding the business aspects of the company.

How to Become an Analyst

Unfortunately, the number of positions for analysts is limited. If you consider that most firms have on average two biotechnology analysts, there are probably no more than 100 biotechnology analyst positions. There are more junior analyst and research associate positions available if you are willing to work for someone else so that you can learn the ropes.

Analyst jobs can be difficult to find. They are not normally advertised in newspapers or in other sources. In addition, research directors usually look for a rare individual with a variety of skills and perhaps some experience in the financial world. To demonstrate that you have the necessary skills, you should be willing to be flexible concerning your expectations.

● ●
"To demonstrate that you have the necessary skills, you should be willing to be flexible concerning your expectations."
● ●

One way to prove yourself is to act as a consultant to an analyst on a special project. You will be paid, you will gain experience in research and writing with the investor in mind, and you will have a product, that is, a report you can use as an example of your work.

You may have to accept a position as a research associate to learn the business. These jobs are not glamorous, and they involve long hours of digging out information for the senior analyst. You could also write some research reports on your own. Pick a company or two that you find interesting, describe the investment potential, and build a financial model for the next few years. This provides you with material to present in an interview that demonstrates your writing skills and your analytical ability. In addition, you can call the investor relations department at the companies you chose to write about and ask them to send you some of the analyst's reports. This will give you an idea of what analyst reports are like.

Because the jobs are not advertised, the best place to start is with current biotechnology analysts. Go to the library and ask for *Nelson's Guide to Institutional Research*. This book lists all of the investments firms, and it gives the names and addresses of all of the analysts. Begin a letter writing campaign. You can start by requesting information, and you can follow up with phone calls for more information: remember that analysts are busy, and they may not return your calls. Be persistent. The key is to be at the right place at the right time, so send your résumé out periodically (every 6 months or so) even if you have not received a response or if you have received a negative response. The landscape is constantly changing as analysts move around and needs change.

There is not really a corporate ladder to climb, unless you start as a research associate or a junior analyst. A research associate helps the analyst do the digging, writes drafts of reports and morning meeting notes, and works on financial models. Research associates also perform certain administrative functions at some firms. Junior analysts typically have a number of small companies that they cover independently, or they may cover companies along with the senior analyst. As the senior analyst, you cover companies on your own. From there, you can be promoted to different levels, depending on the firm, but your duties remain essentially the same.

It is not required that you have a scientific background to be a good analyst; in fact, many analysts do not have a Ph.D. or an M.D. However, I believe that a broad scientific background is very helpful. It is necessary to understand the drug development process, and some scientists are never exposed to this area. Some business experience is also important. You need to be able to converse with business people in their language and to understand their problems. This type of experience can be obtained by getting an M.B.A. and/or by working in the biotechnology or pharmaceutical industry.

The industry experience should also include some involvement in strategic planning or business development, even if it is peripheral to your scientific responsibilities. The goal is to gain some experience in how corporations operate. Scientists sometimes have a tendency not to see the broader picture because they are so involved with the details. It is also helpful to read about companies and the stock market to understand the world you are entering and how your clients—institutional investors—think.

Hence, a combination of skills is required to be a successful biotech analyst. These skills include written and verbal communication skills, scientific and medical knowledge, knowledge of the drug development process, the ability to deal effectively with a diverse group of people, and the ability to rapidly assess the potential of a corporate strategy.

Being a biotech analyst is an exciting and rewarding career. Looking for excellence in companies and watching—sometimes helping—them achieve their goals is gratifying. It is exhilarating to witness the development of whole new areas of medicine that have the potential to revolutionize the way we treat disease.

MY CAREER SINCE SBC WARBURG DILLON READ: MOVING TO THE BUY-SIDE

After several more years as a sell-side analyst, I made the move to the "buy-side." I worked for a large mutual fund and made the decisions for the health care part of the portfolio. This position expanded my job beyond biotechnology because I was required to look at specialty pharmaceutical companies; pharmaceutical companies; health care services companies such as hospitals; HMOs; and laboratory companies. The only health care sector that I did not look at was medical devices because someone else who already covered that area.

The buy-side is challenging because now you are putting your money where your mouth is. You need to evaluate the companies just like a "sell-side" analyst, but since you are covering a broader range of companies, you rely somewhat on sell-side reports to cut down the legwork. In the end, you use all of the available information to make buy and sell decisions on companies in your universe.

The mutual fund that I worked for was somewhat unique because we also invested in private companies. This was a very interesting part of my job. I liked getting to know companies in the early stages of their business and watching them grow. In some cases, I was able to be an observer on the board of directors of these companies. I enjoyed working with boards. I was fortunate to be able to work with some very accomplished people, and I feel that I learned a lot from them. I also felt that my background enabled me to contribute as well.

I enjoyed the board work so much that I eventually decided to make that my career. I am now on the boards of three publicly traded companies: Telik, Inc., Dyax Corp., and Acadia Pharmaceuticals. I have formed a consulting company and also provide consulting services to biotechnology companies. I participate in portfolio and project reviews, as well as other special projects. I also consult for one money management firm. I feel extremely fortunate to be able to control my own destiny and pick and choose the jobs that I take on. I like being more involved with companies and watching the amazing things that small companies are able to do.

THE CORPORATE WORLD

9

....

ENTREPRENEUR AND COMPANY FOUNDER:

Starting Your Own Company and Surviving

. . . .

Ron Cohen, M.D.
CEO and President, Acorda Therapeutics

Although I started out in a medical career, for the past few years I have been creating and building a new biopharmaceutical company, Acorda Therapeutics. The aim of the company is to create novel therapies to treat spinal cord injuries (SCIs) and potentially other neurological damage. Prior to founding Acorda, I was part of the start-up team for Advanced Tissue Sciences, Inc., of San Diego, California. The work of building and growing new companies is hard, but the rewards are great.

My personal goal is to build a company that can develop restorative therapies for SCIs and other neurological damage. I would like to build a model of a company that works efficiently and mobilizes as much of the talent out there as possible to work toward a common goal.

How Did I Get Here?

During my internal medicine residency at the University of Virginia, I saw my first patient with SCI. That experience stayed with me even after I went back to New York City and practiced medicine while pursuing the other love of my

• •
"For a while, I lived a dual life as medical director of a clinic in the Wall Street area and as an ER physician, while also taking acting classes, auditioning and working in commercials, starring in off-off Broadway plays, and appearing as a contestant on Jeopardy.*"*
• •

life—the theater. For a while, I lived a dual life as medical director of a clinic in the Wall Street area and as an ER physician, while also taking acting classes, auditioning and working in commercials, starring in off-off Broadway plays, and appearing as a contestant on *Jeopardy*. I was having a wonderful time, living with one foot in each of two very different worlds.

But then in May 1986, friends from my medical school class at Columbia called and told me about a scientist friend of theirs, Dr. Gail Naughton, who was starting a company that would focus on her work in tissue proliferation. She needed a scientist with an M.D. who was good at making presentations to help build the company. An "acting" M.D. seemed like the perfect solution. My friends had shown Dr. Naughton tapes of me being interviewed for the local news and as a contestant on *Jeopardy*, and she decided that she had found what she was looking for.

I had never considered going into the business world—but this made no difference to Gail. At my first meeting with her, her husband, and her two kids, she pulled out a piece of paper with three lines of writing that essentially said, "I, Ron Cohen, will work for Marrow-Tech for $X," and she said, "Sign here!" While I wanted to think about it, Gail said, "You don't understand. I want you to sign here!" So I did, and that is how I got into biotech—it was an impulse based on the way Gail and I clicked; it just seemed to be the right thing to do.

This simple exchange of "sign here" provided me with the most profound change in my life. Gail and I plunged in without knowing anything about business. A dentist friend of a relative provided the initial money, which ran out after a couple of months. But I was hooked—I worked for no salary and worked part-time in the ER to support myself while Gail was working in the lab at Queensboro Community College to make ends meet.

About 2 years later, we took the company public; recruited a very experienced pharmaceutical executive, Art Benvenuto, as CEO; and grew Marrow-Tech into Advanced Tissue Sciences, Inc., which became a commercial biopharmaceutical firm with approved products entering the marketplace.

A DAY IN THE LIFE OF A CEO

There is no typical day when you head up an early stage company such as Acorda Therapeutics. For the first few years, I was the only full-time employee other than my assistant, so I did anything and everything. The responsibilities of a CEO are overwhelming at times. At this stage in the company's development, raising money is key, along with keeping the "virtual" organization motivated and on track to meet goals. The main responsibilities also include attracting new members of the scientific and business advisory groups who can help the company grow and take things to the next level; planning strategic and financial aspects of the company; accessing new technology for Acorda to develop; and maintaining an intellectual property portfolio. We have to generate and maintain technology licensing agreements, patent applications, research agreements, and corporate partnerships. My assistant, Tierney, now does the in-house financial management and office management, including responding to patients and editing video public relations pieces.

In addition to dealing with company staff, a CEO also must work with the company's board of directors. This group should provide experience and expertise apart from what the in-house management team can provide, it should provide access to networks of potential sources of funding and corporate alliances, and it should critically evaluate the decisions and progress being made by the company. Some of the board members represent groups that have invested heavily in the company.

This means that you have a diverse group of people on the board, each with a different agenda and different past experiences. Managing the board can be a challenge, but a strong, well-balanced board can help a CEO stay ahead of changes in the business and financial environment, and it can allow the CEO to steer the company through rough waters.

The general timetable for each day is about the same, but the activities can be very different. I usually get up at 6:30 A.M. and read the *Wall Street Journal* and the *New York Times*. I head for the office around 8:00 A.M., where I read e-mails and make calls. The rest of the day can be taken up with traveling to meetings with potential investors, potential or existing corporate partners, or scientists whom we wish to recruit; I also attend industry meetings to make contacts. If I am not traveling, the day can include anything from chairing a scientific advisory board (SAB) meeting to conducting a conference call or a meeting to plan a clinical trial program. Each day, I discuss ongoing projects with Acorda's chief scientific officer based in New York and our research director in North Carolina. The day usually ends between 8:00 and 10:00 P.M., with the occasional all-nighter. I work 1 or 2 full days on the weekend, but I try to keep at least half of a day open for fun.

A TYPICAL WORK WEEK

- On Monday, I wrote an ATP grant to apply for $2 million to fund a program, I had a telephone conference on clinical trials, and I worked on financial pro formas (forecasts) with our acting chief financial officer.

- On Tuesday, I flew to an industry meeting in Boston to make a presentation on Acorda as a virtual biotech company, and I had dinner with our chief scientist and our corporate collaborators to discuss the clinical trial program.

- On Wednesday, I attended the rest of the conference and met with a company consultant to discuss corporate development strategies.

- On Thursday, I was back in the office and met with our chief scientist and a potential pharmaceutical partner from Europe. I then met with auditors to get ready for an upcoming audit to prepare for our next financing.

- On Friday, I met with a potential candidate for a full-time chief financial officer position (CFO) and vice president of business development and I had a working session with the acting CFO; I worked on a revision of the executive summary and business plan in preparation for the financing. I went to the chief scientist's lab to discuss recent data, and I worked on a slide show for the financing of the company.

For the next 5 to 10 years, I plan to stay with Acorda and get it to the point where I feel I have accomplished my key goal—successfully developing breakthrough products for restoring neurological functions, which is one of the big remaining frontiers in medicine.

What It Takes to Run the Show

Growing a company from the ground up is definitely "seat-of-the-pants" learning—the first 5 years at Marrow-Tech (which became Advanced Tissue Sciences) were exhilarating and intense, with a series of unremitting crises on a daily basis that often threatened the very survival of the company. This setting is exciting, it requires high adrenaline levels, and it is in certain ways like being at war with buddies. The most exhilarating point came when we lifted our heads out of the trenches and saw that we were actually making progress and building a company.

I became a confirmed adrenaline junkie—which is a good thing. Stress becomes a constant part of your life. Once you take other people's money and are responsible for watching over their investment, everything changes.

"Once you take other people's money and are responsible for watching over their investment, everything changes."

Even more importantly, once you have employees who look to you for their paycheck and health benefits, you realize that your actions impact a wide group of people who depend on you to keep things running. There will always be some crisis or other issue to be resolved. I suggest taking up boxing or racquetball!

Inspiring Others to Work for the Cause

One of the most important skills to have for anyone who is involved in managing a company is the ability to get other people excited and engaged. This is particularly crucial in start-up companies, where a very small team of people works very hard in a very high-risk situation. You have to keep people willing to work long hours for what is frequently low pay. At any given point the company can appear on the threshold of financial or scientific disaster, and the executives at the top have to keep everything moving forward in spite of this. You must be able to motivate folks to take on a broad range of tasks because a young company can't afford to hire enough employees to have specialists.

The CEO had better know exactly what he or she wants to do with the company, what the goals are; then he or she must be able to communicate with others, who must come together to make this goal a reality. Lots of people start companies with the vague idea that they want to be in a certain area of research or clinical development without really having thought through just how to turn that idea into a sustainable business.

You must be able to persuade a group of people from different walks of life—scientists, technology transfer folks at universities, other companies, investors of various types, physicians, lawyers, journalists—that your business is worthwhile. You must enlist their support of your cause.

Communicating with the Public

Communication is the second great task. If you personally are not comfortable communicating in public, you must bring in someone to be the public voice. The CEO doesn't have to be charismatic (although this certainly helps), but someone must be able to communicate clearly about what the company is doing and why it is important. This person must get the outside world excited about the goals. The company lives or dies based on this person's ability to communicate—if outsiders aren't supportive, the company will run out of money and will die before accomplishing anything worthwhile.

You must be able to decide not only what the company's goals are but also how you will implement your decisions and stay on track through inevitable crises. People (employees as well as investors) want to know that the company's leadership is a very clear beacon keeping them off the rocks.

• •
"You must stay the course and keep people optimistic rather than panicky."
• •

You must stay the course and keep people optimistic rather than panicky. As Woody Allen says, 90% of success is just showing up. It takes about a decade for a new pharmaceutical product to move from discovery into the marketplace. The company must survive long enough for an opportunity to come along that you can exploit into a business opportunity. You must be an optimist to keep others fired up. If you are pessimistic, if you constantly look to the possible negative outcomes, why should others persevere?

You need to have the ability to collect and synthesize data, to interview people productively, and to ask the right question at the right time to get the information you need. An important part of my training as an internist was learning how to get a good medical history. A CEO must have the ability to identify people to bring into the company who have the right talent and personality traits, and the CEO must be able to find the right technology to in-license, the right sources of financing, and so forth.

I have found that the ability to identify early on the people who will help you and those who will hurt you is a critical, but apparently rare, skill. Young companies are constantly approached by individuals who portray themselves as "friends and supporters" of the company. But, often, you will find that this friendship lasts only long enough for them to extract whatever they need from you. Sometimes you need to do business with them anyway, but it is always better to know when you are dealing with a real friend and when you are not.

Learn to trust your gut reactions to people and situations, as opposed to overintellectualizing everything. In my experience, in a fight between my gut and my head, my gut is usually right. For example, we have pulled together a scientific advisory board of leading scientists working in different areas related to SCI. Prior to working with Acorda, these folks often competed with each other for grants and publications. As part of our SAB, they work as a team, sharing information and ideas, as well as technology. This requires a strong team spirit and a willingness to work together without betraying the confidence of the group.

My chief scientific officer and I met with a scientist whom we liked immensely and who we thought could provide crucial technical expertise to the SAB. This person elicited a very strong reaction from other scientists in their technical field. Numerous people in the field gave us very negative feedback—it was a real dilemma. But my gut told me that this person was important for achieving the ultimate goal. I went with my gut feeling. Now 3 years later, this decision has shown itself to be one of my best ones. This person is one of the key performers on the team and a real asset to others on the team. Had we gone with our heads, we would have made the wrong decision.

This gut instinct will be important when making decisions about potential corporate partners, bankers, and employees. In addition, young companies tend to use consultants to help handle some of the more specialized tasks, such as business development, financial analysis of deal points, corporate communications with the press and the financial community, clinical and regulatory affairs, and manufacturing. Because these folks are working outside of the company, you need to identify those folks who really have your best interests at heart and who are conscientious and honest.

THE PROS AND CONS OF BEING THE BOSS

- **What I like the most:** I enjoy building teams of extraordinary individuals to do extraordinary things. It is a rush to get a group of very talented and motivated people of good will to come together to do something challenging and worthy. And we are all working toward goals that we can be very proud of in a humane sense. This is the best of all worlds.

- **What I like the least:** Invariably, our progress in the science exceeds our ability to fund the work. I am impatient and hate the time needed to raise money. Biotech firms never seem to have sufficient funds to implement fully their strategic plan, to build the team as fast as they want. This means that I have to spend an inordinate amount of time gathering the capital until the company is able to fund itself. This is particularly true in biotech because the product development path is long (7 to 10 years), and it takes years to get a product to market and generate significant revenues.

  One of the problems with running a lean machine is that the money limits how many employees the company has and what they are paid for working in a very high-risk environment. I didn't receive a salary for the first 3 years. Instead, I worked for a significant chunk of founders' stock, which will some day be very valuable if we make Acorda a success. Recently, the board voted that I receive an annual salary of $120,000, based on the closing of our first corporate deal and the company having made sufficient progress and having raised sufficient funding.

HOW CAN YOU GET THIS JOB?

These start-up positions are not usually advertised. You generate the opportunity yourself by starting a company, or you find someone who has just started a company and join their team to learn the process (as I did with Advanced Tissue Sciences).

I founded Acorda from scratch and on my own dime. This meant several years of deciding which area I wanted the company to pursue; plowing through the technical literature and attending scientific and clinical conferences to find out the current status of SCI research and therapeutic development; identifying the top scientists in the field and persuading them to work with me; figuring out what the other biopharmaceutical companies were doing in the area; and getting the various not-for-profit foundations that fund SCI research to cooperate with us rather than compete. Then I had to write a business plan that made scientific, clinical, commercial, and financial sense. Hardest of all, I had to round up sufficient investment dollars to fund the company. This last task never ends, but you won't have a company without the first infusion of dollars.

If you want to become involved with someone else's company, you have to use your network to reach the main job contact at the company. Start with people you know who are already in the industry or are leading scientists in the field. For example, the best way to find out about opportunities in a start-up working on new drugs to treat Alzheimer's disease is to identify and network with the scientists who are developing key technology in that field.

Keep your ears open—if there is a talk being given by someone from a company, go and meet that person and network—this is a critical skill if you want to get into business. If any of your friends or professors have contacts in the relevant arena, make sure you network with them and express enthusiasm and interest.

What about entrepreneurs who come right out of academia? In a strange way, ignorance of the business world can be useful for entrepreneurs. One of the hardest things anyone could ever do is to start his or her own company. Had I known just how hard it really would be to get Advanced Tissue Sciences up and rolling, I might have been scared off. The advantage is to be naïve—we were too ignorant to know we could possibly not succeed. Once we were committed, we just struggled to keep our heads above water. It was the hardest, yet most exciting thing I had ever done.

At some point, however, experience is crucial. My Acorda experience is very challenging—huge amounts of work and stress, but at least I knew what was coming. I strongly urge budding entrepreneurs to ally themselves with people who do have that experience, to balance out their ignorance. Scientists need to align themselves with people with management and people skills, those who have been through it before. This requires swallowing your ego. It is hard to share control with others, but often it is a fatal mistake for entrepreneurs to try and go at it alone. Strong scientific skills do not translate directly into excellence in other areas. A Nobel laureate does not necessarily make a good CEO.

THE CURRENT SITUATION

In 2003 to 2004, Acorda weathered two significant setbacks, one a decision by some of its investors not to accept a $45 million initial public offering and the other a disappointing result in two pivotal trials of its lead drug candidate for SCI. We promptly set out to acquire a commercial product for our therapeutic area and succeeded in bringing in Zanaflex, an approved drug for spasticity due to SCI, a multiple sclerosis (MS) stroke, and other central nervous system injuries. We are now generating revenue from this drug, and we have built our initial sales and marketing organization. In 2005, Acorda has 59 employees and, in addition to Zanaflex, a drug product that is about to enter Phase 3 of a pivotal trial for restoration of function in MS. We have additional, exciting pipeline products that have been shown to repair nerve pathways in the spinal cord and brain of animal models. The company has raised more than $140 million since inception, mostly from venture capital groups. Biotechnology companies underscore (perhaps more than most) the need to have management teams that are creative and opportunistic at every turn, allowing the companies to come through the inevitable setbacks successfully.

Chapter

10

·········

BUSINESS DEVELOPMENT:

Making Deals with Science

●●●●●●●●●●●●●●●●●

Ronald Pepin, Ph.D.

Senior Vice President, Business Development, Medarex, Inc.

MY EVOLUTION

I didn't plan to leave the lab and become a deal maker. It just sort of happened. After busting my hump at lab benches next to autoclaves, after labeling an infinite number of Eppendorf tubes for endless sequencing reactions, after a variety of battles with ^{32}P, after extraordinary moments of joy with successful experiments and new hope after failures, I never planned to throw in the lab coat and its associated rewards for a tie. It just happened. Suddenly, I was dealing in the millions of dollars instead of plaques, telling people about the merits and flaws of their research from a commercial instead of a scientific perspective, and wading through buckets of biotech hype. And, to quote Maxwell Smart, "Loving it!"

As a molecular biologist with a Ph.D., I had been at the bench for a couple of biotech companies before I decided that I had been here and done that—once you have cloned a few genes, the excitement can wear off, especially when they now make kits for all the cutting-edge work I used to perform! Before I traded in my pipette man for a Mont Blanc pen, I had no idea what was involved in business development.

Even as a researcher at a small biotech company where everyone knew each other and their functions quite well, the business development guys were just part of the typical biotech "dog and pony show" that was constantly staged to keep the company afloat and me with a paycheck. Quite honestly, as with most jobs, you really don't know what it is all about until you do it. I was pleasantly surprised to find my true calling.

WHAT IS BUSINESS DEVELOPMENT?

Business development involves the exchange of items either into or out of your company to enhance your company's business. The items that are commonly exchanged can be intellectual property (e.g., patents or patent applications), technologies, know-how, compounds, drugs, research collaborations, equity investments in a company, and so on. The broad scope of the transactions that can be completed make the job both challenging and exciting. The exchange of these items can be done on an exclusive (for one company only) or nonexclusive (shared by two or more parties) basis. Financially, the transactions to accomplish your exchange may involve the simple exchange of money or may involve the transfer of goods, property, ideas, or other creative means that ensure that both parties obtain what they want and need.

I have had the fortunate experience of seeing the world of business development from both sides of the coin. My business development career started with a large, multinational pharmaceutical company ("big pharma"), Bristol-Myers Squibb. Like most big pharmas, BMS is a profitable company with broad interests and sales, spanning small molecule drugs, as well as biotherapeutics. I eventually moved on and joined a biotechnology firm (in the "biotech" arena), Medarex , which is much more focused, specializing in the commercialization of fully human monoclonal antibodies.

Business development at a biotech company usually means that you sell and out-license your technology and/or products more than you in-license. My experience at Medarex has been uniquely satisfying in that I do a mix of both. Medarex is a biotech company with a proprietary platform technology for making fully human monoclonal antibodies in transgenic mice. To most fully capitalize in commercializing this powerful platform, Medarex has strategically decided to make the technology broadly available to large pharmaceutical and biotech companies, as well as to use it for generating its own proprietary products. To get the platform into experienced drug discovery companies, Medarex engaged in what we call "cash and carry deals." In return for licensing fees, upfront payments, milestones and royalties, we will ship our transgenic mice to a partner so that they can raise antibodies in the mice for their own development within their organization. This allows us to generate revenue at very little cost from the world-class platform that we have generated (at a higher cost). Thus, out-licensing is an important part of our corporate strategy.

To generate our product pipeline by using the mouse platform, we access novel, validated drug targets from a variety of sources: universities, government agencies, and other biotech companies. In the latter case, we often work with genomic and proteomic companies that specialize in identifying new potential targets but that do not have the internal expertise or infrastructure to generate potential drugs against these novel targets. In such cases, we forge an alliance based on equal sharing: they supply the target, we make a human antibody against the target, and we share costs and profits on bringing this discovery to the market. By signing a large number of these 50/50 partnerships, we have assembled a strong internal pipeline in collaboration with our partners. These in-licensing deals help us to execute our pipeline strategy. Being a smaller company with a streamlined decision-making process and having a smaller number of decision makers, we can accomplish deals quickly and can demonstrate a great deal of flexibility.

Big Pharma Biz Dev

In contrast to my biotech experience, business development at Bristol-Myers Squibb was usually a one-way flow of in-licensing technology and products into the company. To best perform this broad overarching function, business development was divided among several different groups, each of which had its own niche. This also allowed each group to have particular expertise among its members. As a part of the research division, the External Science and Technology (EST) group was responsible for the acquisition of early stage technology from biotech companies, universities, and government agencies on a worldwide basis. The deals that this group performed range from simple licenses to drug discovery targets, receptors, or other forms of intellectual property, up to extensive research collaborations with biotech companies, which typically included up-front payments, licensing fees, research funding, payments for the achievement of clinical milestones, and royalty payments. The deals could have also included an equity investment in the stock of the biotech company, which involves the valuation of the company and its platform technologies.

To complement the work of EST, a second business development group focused on the licensing compounds that were in clinical development. The agreements put together by this group were similar in structure to EST deals (i.e., up-front licensing fees, research support in some cases, clinical milestone payments, and royalties on product sales). Some deals also involved an equity investment. The client group of this licensing team, however, was broader than just the drug discovery division of research. Much more attention was paid to financial projections. Because the compound and its potential indication use have been identified, the market projections for such a drug are more predictable than something in early preclinical research as a part of one of EST's research alliances. The licensing group would also interact more extensively with the clinical division, which had a justifiably heavy influence on the licensing deal. Marketing considerations were also more important for these later-stage deals.

The mission of EST was to enhance the ability of the research group to discover new drug candidates. The job involved both the proactive and reactive evaluation of technology to match its fit with the needs of the research division of BMS. On the proactive front, EST visited universities, government agencies, and biotech companies to learn the novel technologies that they had uncovered and, if available, to evaluate their value to BMS. Alternative proactive approaches included attending scientific meetings, partnering conferences, and investment banker meetings to track down the sources that are discovering cutting-edge technology. Such "one-stop mall shopping" is a time- and cost-effective way to survey multiple opportunities in a short period of time and to build one's mental database of the playing field in the business.

In addition to the excitement of proactive prospecting for appropriate opportunities, EST and other business development professionals had to react to unsolicited proposals. We received on the order of 800 to 1000 proposals per year from any university technology transfer agent or biotech business development representative worth their salt. EST personnel served as a first screen of such proposals. It was our responsibility to filter out and reject the real turkeys (I have received nonconfidential data on alien spaceship warp drives, no kidding!) and to discuss with the appropriate scientists within the organization the technologies that have substance and merit and that may fit the company's research strategy.

Once a technology was identified as one in which BMS indeed had an interest, we quickly started to move matters ahead. If the initial disclosure about the technology was nonconfidential in nature (i.e., a very brief and usually rather uninformative document designed to whet our appetite for the technology), we would request to see confidential information under the rules and regulations of a Confidential Disclosure Agreement, or CDA. A CDA is a legal document designed to protect the disclosing party from having their confidential intellectual property (such as a novel cloned gene) from being plagiarized by the people who view the documents.

If the confidential data package (with an emphasis on the existence of data) still looked impressive, BMS would invite the scientists who made the discovery to make a scientific presentation to the in-house scientists. The business development person would attend such sessions to learn about the proposed technology so that he or she could help value the information for BMS and formulate a deal strategy to bring the technology into BMS.

The Art of Negotiation

At this point, a commitment needed to be made by both sides. If there was interest from both parties to move ahead and strike a deal, then the proper structure for the interaction needed to be formulated. Both sides also had to negotiate in good faith such that if a "win-win" agreement could be reached, both parties would execute it. I was involved in negotiating major proposed alliances where BMS moved forward in good faith, only to have the other party decline on doing the deal at the eleventh hour. One actual deal was closer to 11:59 P.M.—I had a huge equity investment and R&D alliance being voted on by the BMS board of directors, only to find out that the other party had been negotiating with several parties at the same time!

I have also worked with skilled professionals who know their job and the value of their technology. Such individuals make the negotiation process as painless as possible. Most people would assume that I would rather work with a rookie negotiator of whom I could take advantage. In reality, it is much more difficult to negotiate with someone who has no knowledge of what is included in a typical contract and what terms are the norm for the industry for a given type of deal and technology. It is about the same as teaching your surgeon how to operate during your heart transplant. It just seems to go more smoothly if they have been there before!

In any event, the most exciting component of the deal revolves around the negotiation. To those who have not been there, it would appear that once the horse-trading over money is completed, the negotiations are over. But, nooooooo! Now the lawyers enter the mix! That means that the good old English language has to be put into "legalese" before it becomes a final, unambiguous document. And getting there, if you ever do, is the most laborious, time-consuming part of the whole process.

•••••••••••••••••••••
"To those who have not been there, it would appear that once the horse-trading over money is completed, the negotiations are over. But, nooooooo! Now the lawyers enter the mix!"
•••••••••••••••••••••

In all seriousness, the lawyers play an important and helpful role for both negotiating parties by crafting language that will protect their respective clients. It is just that the dotting of the *i*s and crossing of the *t*s can be a painful experience. Each party usually has its own sensitivities that need to be recognized and met by the other negotiating party. And some sensitivities are more sensitive than others!

You have to pick your battles and go to the mat on the most important issues, while your ability and need to compromise must arise on some other lesser issues to make the negotiation work. Holding your ground on each and every point will only serve to kill the deal. Even if you are the party with the "upper hand" (i.e., you have the money), you simply cannot insist on your way on every issue if you want to complete a deal that is favorable to both sides. My personal philosophy is that if both parties leave the negotiation table feeling good but with some bad taste in their mouth, the negotiation was a success.

SOME OF THE CHALLENGES

The external negotiations (i.e., those with the third party with whom you are doing the deal) on any alliance are often easier than the internal negotiation process that must take place within your own company to sell the deal. The internal selling of a deal involves the buy-in of many diverse groups of people beyond the original scientists who became excited by the deal: financial analyzers, legal professionals, the tax department, and other business development groups, not to mention management at all levels. Because these groups have different backgrounds and are not commonly trained as scientists, the ability to translate complex scientific concepts into lay language becomes an important skill to possess for this job. I view it as the innate ability to teach. Just remember back to graduate school where the hotshot research professors were generally the very worst at explaining and spreading their knowledge to students.

If you want to sell your deal, you better know not only the scientific complexities but also ways to convey the financial importance to your organization's management! Use graphs, figures, analogies, and anything that will convince those who control the purse strings that the deal is truly important for your company. This also is true for the small companies and universities trying to sell the technology. Their internal sell job is somewhat different

• •
"If you want to sell your deal, you better know not only the scientific complexities but also ways to convey the financial importance to your organization's management!"
• •

because it is generally easier to sell someone on accepting money rather than on spending it. However, since most biotech and university managers are trained scientists rather than business people, you probably have to provide similar data on the fairness of the deal: benchmark it against other similar deals, and demonstrate the value to your organization to make it fly. The financial gurus will provide you with estimates of the market value of the products that may arise from the alliance, which will be an important concept to relay to your business-focused management. And, of course, they will want to see that the legal and tax divisions have given the contract a seal of approval.

If an equity investment is involved, a detailed explanation of the price per share that you are paying to a biotech company will be required. Here is one area where experience in the industry will really pay off. It is easy to value a publicly traded biotech company, but producing a valuation for a private company is an art form. It involves evaluation of its "platform technologies," comparisons to comparables, and its previous financing.

By factoring in all these variables and the level of interest your company has in doing such an investment, you can arrive at a price that is acceptable to both parties. Your management may, however, take some comfort in having your valuation backed up by an external evaluation firm. In any case, you can always protect your investment against any pumped-up price sought by the biotech company by instituting antidilution provisions in the equity document. These provisions allow you to make an investment at a set price, but they guarantee that the company in which you invest will not sell additional shares to another party at a price lower than that paid by your company. If they do sell off cheaper shares, the antidilution provisions spell out how the company will compensate you for that transaction (e.g., they can give you additional shares to make you whole on your investment such that you pay the same lower price paid by someone else).

WHAT YOU NEED TO SUCCEED IN BUSINESS DEVELOPMENT

A typical day in business development involves a great deal of communication. Large phone bills and long hours at the keyboard answering e-mails are "par for the course." Given that you may spend anywhere from 10% to 75% of your time traveling, the business development executive commonly may be found doing the above-mentioned communication on the road!

If oral and written communication skills are not your strength, stay away from business development! And shy introverts need not apply. You will be eaten alive at the negotiation table if you don't like to speak up and counteract your counterpart sitting across from you. The art of negotiation can take several different forms, ranging from bluffing to putting all your cards on the table. The key in my mind is to be honest and fair and to negotiate in good faith, with true interest in striking a deal.

"If oral and written communication skills are not your strength, stay away from business development!"

One thing that initially attracted me to the business development field was the unique opportunity it affords a scientist to make use of his or her hard-earned degree in the sciences. In addition, it allows you to play a part in the business aspects of your company or university. My experience (bias?) has taught me that it is easier for a Ph.D.-trained scientist to pick up the business aspects of this job than it is for a person with an M.B.A. to pick up on the subtleties of the science. After all, we all have to balance our checkbooks and negotiate for cars. On the other hand, how many of your nonscientist friends have ever done a Northern Blot? Analytical skills are needed to fairly, quickly, and accurately evaluate a vast variety of scientific proposals, to uncover new research opportunities, and to analyze the business aspects of a deal.

> *"My experience (bias?) has taught me that it is easier for a Ph.D.-trained scientist to pick up the business aspects of this job than it is for a person with an M.B.A. to pick up on the subtleties of the science."*

I feel privileged to have seen the biotechnology field from both sides of the coin: from the lab bench and sell-side of a biotech company to the wheeling and dealing as part of business development at a large pharmaceutical company. I believe that this past gives me the perspective to see how different aspects of a deal are important to different parties and how it is vital to satisfy the major needs of both parties. It has added to my ability to be creative in structuring alliances that are workable for both sides of the agreement.

How Do You Get Here?

Getting into this racket is not necessarily easy. Most large companies and biotech firms justifiably require that you have experience before they will hire you. That said, one way to join the ranks of business development is to work at the lab bench within a company so that you develop a strong positive reputation. Such a "known quantity" can parlay that reputation to gain the confidence of company management and to secure a business development position.

I would rather train a competent scientist from within my company who possesses other desirable personal and professional characteristics than to hire an individual from the outside about whom I know very little (how much do you really learn in a 1-hour interview?). This allows me to mold these scientists in such a way that they perform their business development duties in a manner and style of which I approve.

I also have a strong bias toward making these choice opportunities available first to people who work in my company. Given the small size of this function within most companies, you must choose and develop your team very carefully to be effective!

An alternate mechanism for joining the business development club is to pay your dues at a university technology transfer office rather than working your way up via the bench. Most major universities have an office that employs individuals who are responsible for the out-licensing of university technology to large and small companies. Because universities generally pay less money, and the deals are most often less complicated in structure than biotech deals with big pharma, this is a prime training ground for learning this trade.

A few years of experience in this environment gives you the training to make the leap to an industrial position. Once you have completed some deals at a biotech or pharmaceutical company, you join the elite few business development people who actually have experience in the field. At that point, you can write your own ticket. You will find that the headhunters, the best source of such positions outside of word of mouth, will be calling you on a regular basis! Salaries for novices in the industry fall in the range of $90,000 to $100,000 (again, universities pay less) and seasoned professionals can make well in excess of six figures.

In conclusion, a position in business development gives you the opportunity to use your scientific training and creativity without being anchored to the lab bench. It provides the opportunity to travel, to attend scientific and business conferences, to learn about the business aspects of the pharmaceutical industry, to explore scientific areas well outside of those on which your research focused, and to make new acquaintances in one of the most fascinating industries available to you as a scientist. Although the business may on a few rare occasions frustrate the hell out of you, the rewards far exceed the negatives. Now go out there and do a deal!

11

· · · · · · · · · ·

THE GROWTH OF A MANAGER:

From Pure Research to Policy Administration

· · · · · · · · · · · · · · · · ·

Philip W. Hammer, Ph.D.

Vice President, The Franklin Center, Franklin Institute Science Museum
Former Director of the Society of Physics Students and Assistant Director
of the Education Division, American Institute of Physics

What is a Ph.D., and what is it good for? To the "zeroth order," as physicists would say, the Ph.D., or doctor of philosophy, is a scholarly degree that trains people in scientific inquiry and research. The student also learns to write and speak in the course of presenting and defending his or her findings. Occasionally, some teaching experience is thrown in. Hence, the Ph.D. is designed to qualify a person to work in academia as a scholar doing research and preparing the next generation of those pursuing Ph.D.s.

Given this information, many are surprised to learn that fewer than 8% of those with a bachelor's degree in physics actually end up filling this Ph.D.-to-academia career niche. The other 92% land in a range of professions as varied as the individuals holding the physicist's sheepskin. I am one of those in the 92%. Although I earned my Ph.D. at a prestigious university, studying under a respected advisor and then proceeding to a post-doctoral fellowship in one of the most competitive groups in my field, I went on to work as the assistant manager of the Education Division at the American Institute of Physics (AIP). I am now vice president of the Franklin Center at the Franklin Institute Science Museum.

WHAT IS ORGANIZATION MANAGEMENT?

What qualified me for my job in organization management? First and foremost, according to the job description, was that the applicant must have a Ph.D. in physics. That was simple, but what is it about managing a group that runs physics education programs that makes the Ph.D. necessary?

The primary answer has to do with communication. Besides training for research, studying to obtain the Ph.D. is also a socialization process whereby one becomes a member of a community with common traditions, mores, and ways of communicating. To be effective in the physics community and to have credibility, a person should be a part of the physics culture. It is not necessary, of course, but it is beneficial and substantially improves that person's ability to communicate and empathize with physicists as physicists.

The second item on the job description stated that the applicant must have considerable experience as a physics educator. This was problematic for me because the extent of my teaching background was as a teaching assistant in graduate school. To get the job, I would therefore have to persuade the people doing the hiring that I would bring other qualities and experiences to the division that would mitigate my lack of teaching experience.

At this point, it may be instructive to elaborate on what the AIP Education Division does. Its primary job is to run the Society of Physics Students (SPS) and Sigma Pi Sigma. SPS is a professional society, primarily for undergraduate physics students, with about 6000 members. Sigma Pi Sigma is the physics honor society, with about 35,000 members. Running these two organizations requires managing staff and coordinating the range of services provided for our members.

In addition to administering these two organizations, our division published a hands-on science magazine and an electronic physics education newsletter; we were also initiating new programs to serve physics students and educators. Thus, to manage this group effectively requires experience in administration, management, organization, and also vision and ideas about the division's future and its role within the physics community and society. It was my professional experience after my post-doc that added the real value to my Ph.D. and qualified me for this job.

• • • • • • • • • • • • • • • • • • • •

"It was my professional experience after my post-doc that added the real value to my Ph.D. and qualified me for this job."

• • • • • • • • • • • • • • • • • • • •

HOW DID THIS HAPPEN TO ME?

Near the end of my post-doc, I decided that I should expand my career options by getting experience in science policy. This decision was motivated by my apprehension about increasing competition in the academic job market and by my own interests in policy and the role of science in society.

While reading *Physics Today*, I learned about the Congressional Science Fellows program and the physicists who became fellows. During the next couple of years, I became increasingly intrigued with the idea of applying to the program. Discussions on the Young Scientists Network and my own perceptions of the world in 1993 catalyzed my decision to go for it. On my birthday that year, I got the call telling me that I had been selected by the American Physical Society to be one of their two fellows for the 1993–1994 class.

Congressional fellows are sponsored by a large number of professional societies. The program is designed to bring scientific expertise into the legislative process, while simultaneously exposing the science community to the intricacies of how policy is made at the federal level. Fellows spend a year on the staff of either a member of Congress or a congressional committee.

Ostensibly, fellows are brought in to be the staff science expert. In reality, they become integrated into the staff mix and work on a variety of issues, few of which have science content. I chose to work for the House Science Committee, so my immersion in science policy was greater than that of many others in my class. My year on Capitol Hill left me poised to make a career transition into science policy and management.

• •
"My year on Capitol Hill left me poised to make a career transition into science policy and management."
• •

My next move was into another post-doctoral type of position, only this time it was not in science or policy but in management. Again, an ad in *Physics Today* caught my eye. This job was dubbed "Physics Management Fellow," a temporary position designed to train a young physicist in management while serving as an assistant to the executive director of AIP. This job was a natural transition from the congressional fellowship, and it honed my writing, speaking, management, and negotiating skills.

More important, being a physics management fellow was an opportunity to positively impact an organization in which there were opportunities for professional growth into permanent positions. Or, it could be a good launching point into a permanent policy or management position elsewhere.

When the education job opened up 2 years later, I was in a very good position to apply. My main challenge was to persuade AIP that the diversity of my background would compensate for my lack of direct experience as an educator. My 2 years in the director's office allowed me to gain the confidence of AIP management and demonstrate my abilities. Had I applied from the outside, I probably would not have been successful.

WHAT DOES A POLICY ADMINISTRATOR DO ALL DAY?

After landing the education job, I had a whole new set of challenges and skills to learn. I quickly learned that my job basically had two components— daily administration and management of long-term projects—that require different ways of thinking and different rates of energy expenditure.

Administration is a high-wattage activity, requiring lots of motion and human interaction. In contrast, projects get done at more of a slow burn, with much intellectual energy expended in the process of developing ideas and making plans. Working on projects is a lot like research in terms of the creativity and thought involved, while the challenge in administration is to work with the division's management team to motivate staff and to coordinate the big picture of activities. My biggest challenge in this job was learning to make the transition between administration and project management efficiently so that my productivity did not crash.

Outreach was a major component of my job. It was very important that our division be visible and accessible to our constituents. This meant a lot of time on the phone and e-mail, and it also meant much travel around the country to visit schools and attend conferences. During the academic year, I probably averaged about one 4-day trip per month. On many of these trips, I gave talks, and each trip required varying levels of summary reports. Travel, including preparation and wrap-up, was a time-consuming but critical component of the job.

My job was professionally rewarding for many reasons. I got credit and recognition for the work I did, both within AIP in terms of advancement and within the physics community in terms of professional visibility from talks and publications. Professional recognition is particularly important because, although I no longer make scientific contributions to physics, I made contributions in advancing physics and physicists as a professional community.

As noted earlier, I spent considerable time on outreach tasks, either writing articles or traveling to give talks. My activity became focused on assessing the relationship between physics and society with particular attention paid to the undergraduate degree and its perceived lack of usefulness to students. Specifically, I was concerned that the 38-year low in the number of undergraduate degrees in physics was an indicator that students and employers no longer viewed physics as a useful course of study.

In my travels and writing, I attempted to persuade students and the physics faculty that physics (or science in general, for that matter) was the best training for a professional life in our technical society and that, as a professional community, we should aggressively promote this notion to students and the public.

COMPARING THE WORK

The work style in my job was intense but steady for 8 to 9 hours per day. This, coupled with my ability to make daily progress on important projects, was satisfying and suitable to my lifestyle because I was able to advance professionally and still have time for life outside of work. My hours and my ability to make progress were also different in comparison to my previous jobs.

Research could be managed in a normal day, but there was always a subtext of pressure stemming from possible competition from another lab and from making progress in the name of next year's funding proposal. The upside of research, and its similarity to my job, was that the ideas and outcomes had my name on them, making my performance measurable and recognizable as my output.

In Congress, I worked hard on important issues, and from a congressional perspective, I made significant contributions. For example, in the subcommittee for which I worked, we labored for about 9 months on a bill to reauthorize high energy and nuclear physics in the aftermath of Congress's killing of the Superconducting Super Collider (SSC). Our bill was eventually passed by the House of Representatives. As with all House-passed bills, this one moved over to the Senate for approval; due to timing, it died a slow death by neglect.

This is a typical story in Congress: people work very hard to craft legislation, yet relatively few bills are signed into law. The legislative process is slow and incremental, and while this may be part of the genius of our system of government, it can be frustrating for the individuals who want to see their hard work pay off maximally.

On the other hand, even though our bill never became law, the policy it laid out did have a lasting effect. The death of the SSC forced high-energy physicists to work with Congress and the Executive Branch in setting priorities for the future of their field. This cooperation and the way in which the scientists formulated their recommendations resulted in a generous bump in funding that helped keep high-energy physics healthy during the post-SSC transition. In this instance, scientists working with Congress and the federal agencies crafted a rational national science policy.

Another frustrating factor about working in Congress is that most creative output, such as speeches and Op-Ed pieces, is perceived as the work of a member of Congress, not the staff person who actually crafted the words. At AIP, meaningful progress on issues that affect real people could be made daily, and I got credit for my work.

What's Next?

Few career trajectories are deterministic. As a college student in my first physics class, I had no vision of myself sitting in College Park 12 years later worrying about the state of physics education. I do not think that an undergraduate can plot a strategy for becoming assistant manager of the education division of an organization. The process is too nonlinear and dependent on timing and the relationships between individuals to have an outcome that can be predetermined.

My career strategy in college was to proceed in a manner that kept my options as open as possible. After receiving my B.S., getting a Ph.D. seemed like the natural next step in keeping with this strategy. In retrospect, this was a wise decision because of the intense "professionalization" that occurs in the Ph.D. process.

Similarly, the unpredictability of career planning also applies to questions of where I go from here. For a scientist with experience in policy and management, there are many organizations in the Washington, D.C. area that could provide good opportunities. Within any one organization, such as AIP, the opportunities for advancement exist but occur less frequently.

For those desiring a career in nonprofit management in a science-related organization, I would suggest that being a member of the represented community is key, which suggests the need for a Ph.D. However, while probably necessary, a Ph.D. is not sufficient. Growth and experience in nonscience areas, such as management or policy, are important for developing the worldview, maturity, and temperament required for the position.

What is the Ph.D. good for? The Ph.D. is good training for a professional life. For me, it was my entrée into the culture of physics and the first step to my current job. This argument only works after the fact, however. Others at AIP have landed their jobs via a different route than I, but among the physicists, the post-B.S. study is our common bond.

Update: 7 Years Later

In 2000, I left the American Institute of Physics after being recruited to join the staff of The Franklin Institute Science Museum in Philadelphia as vice president for the Franklin Center. Much about what qualified me for my position at AIP was what caught the attention of The Franklin Institute: a Ph.D. in physics, nonprofit management experience, good contacts in the science community, focus on science education and policy, and ability to adapt professionally.

In many ways, my work at The Franklin Institute (TFI) is similar to what I did at AIP: I essentially manage a series of programs that are driven by mission. However, TFI is completely different from AIP in audience, revenue, geographic focus, and mission. AIP is a professional society designed to serve the broadly defined international physics community. Revenue comes primarily from the sale of scholarly journals. TFI is a cultural institution with a science education mission. The audience is mostly local children and their families or teachers—about 1 million of them per year, each buying an admission ticket at some full or discounted price. Most revenue is earned or raised person-by-person and donor-by-donor. The rest comes from grants and endowment. Thus, most of the effort is focused on delivering a "product" to our customers, whether it be new permanent exhibits or traveling exhibits, live floor programs, IMAX films, Web-based educational resources, and related outreach programs.

My particular responsibilities are the Franklin Medals and Bower Awards (a venerable science and engineering awards program dating back to the 1820s), the *Journal of The Franklin Institute* (a science and engineering journal first published in 1826!), and the institute's library and collections (which include Benjamin Franklin and Wright Brothers materials, as well as numerous other historical treasures). Running the awards program has many similarities to what I did at AIP; indeed, this is why I was hired. However, managing a journal, a library, and overseeing the institute's collections also came with the Franklin Center's territory, and this is where I have learned an incredible amount and expanded my skill set. Collections, and the exhibits and programs they enhance, are at the core of any museum's mission. Thus, I have had the great fortune to be able to now call myself a "museum professional," as well as a physicist.

Yes, few career trajectories are deterministic, and the only thing a person can accurately predict about the future is that it is unpredictable. I would be disappointed if this pattern did not continue in some fashion.

Chapter

12

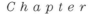

REGULATORY AFFAIRS:

Keeping Product Development on Track

Elizabeth D. Moyer, Ph.D.

CEO, M/P Biomedical Consultants, LLC

Former Senior Vice President of Product Development, Kinetek Pharmaceuticals, Inc.

In the world of shrinking numbers of research grants and funding and fewer academic positions, there is a drive to find less traditional careers in science. In the last few years, there has been a dramatic decrease in NIH grants awarded to scientists under the age of 36 years.

Michael Teitelbaum of the Sloane Foundation, speaking at a National Research Council public meeting on trends in early research careers of life scientists, asked in the open forum whether it would make a difference to entering graduate students if they knew that they only had a 10% to 20% chance of obtaining an academic research position. Clearly, to some it would, but at the same time, this partly reflects the intellectual environment in academic training.

Many academic faculties have a negative attitude toward nontraditional career paths. In fact, early in my career I was told by one department head at a major university that only students headed toward an academic profession were considered for the graduate program.

Current science training also does not direct students toward nontraditional career paths. Generally, the "best" students are steered toward graduate school and then on to an academic career, with little discussion of the other available options. A visible pathway does not exist for young scientists who would like to choose less traditional careers.

One such alternate pathway is that of regulatory affairs. People go into regulatory affairs for about the same list of reasons people go into science itself. Some just want a job, some have more altruistic reasons (e.g., making a difference, helping people), and some are drawn into it and find it rewarding for various personal, intellectual, and professional reasons.

For a scientist, even one without an advanced degree, this field represents a reasonable career alternative to the grant-restricted world of academic science. In addition to using the philosophy ingrained as part of scientific training, specific skills and interests gained during college, graduate school, and/or post-doctoral work can also be critical.

• •
"For a scientist, even one without an advanced degree, this field represents a reasonable career alternative to the grant-restricted world of academic science."
• •

While regulatory affairs can affect the quality of the food you eat, the cosmetics you apply, or the medicines you take, in this chapter I will focus most specifically on regulatory affairs as it applies to the pharmaceutical industry.

WHAT IS REGULATORY AFFAIRS?

As a discipline, regulatory affairs covers a broad range of specific skills and occupations. Under the best of circumstances, it is composed of a group of people who act as a liaison between the potentially conflicting worlds of government, industry, and consumers to help make sure that marketed products are safe and effective when used as advertised. People who work in regulatory affairs negotiate the interaction between the regulators (the government), the regulated (industry), and the market (consumers) to get good products to the market and to keep them there while preventing bad products from being sold.

The range of products covered is enormous, including foods and agricultural products, veterinary products, surgical equipment and medical devices, *in vitro* and *in vivo* diagnostic tools and tests, and drugs (which range from small molecules to proteins). The range of issues addressed is huge, such as manufacturing and analytical testing, preliminary safety and efficacy testing, clinical trials, and postmarketing follow-up. Advertising issues, with a healthy dose of data management, document preparation, project management, budgeting, issue negotiation, and conflict resolution, are thrown in the mix.

Over the years, a complicated system of checks and balances has developed to set in place a process to efficiently and effectively regulate the marketing of products. On the industry side, people in regulatory affairs work with research scientists, clinicians, manufacturing groups, and sales and marketing groups to make sure that the government has the information it needs to judge a product. On the government side, people in regulatory affairs work to interpret and implement laws that Congress establishes to help protect the public. To carry out the congressional mandate, the Food and Drug Administration (FDA) requires pharmaceutical companies to generate and provide all the information deemed necessary to evaluate a given drug, biologic, and/or device with respect to safety and efficacy. This information is used by the agency to decide whether the product should be on the market—and if so, how it should be marketed and sold.

On the consumer side, people in regulatory affairs help keep the other two groups honest, and they provide the stimulus for Congress to enact the laws that regulate how government and industry treat products.

REGULATORY AFFAIRS IN A BIOPHARMACEUTICAL COMPANY

Typical functions of a regulatory affairs group in a pharmaceutical company include interacting with regulatory authorities, preparing documents for regulatory submission, developing regulatory strategies, and interacting with company staff. Each of these responsibilities can have major implications on the success or failure of the company.

Interacting with the government is a crucial role within the company that is frequently restricted to the regulatory group. Whenever a company contacts the government, both sides typically document all topics discussed and the issues raised and answered. Funneling all conversations through the regulatory group prevents different people from making commitments to the government that are not fully known by the rest of the company. Typical topics for discussion include the following:

- The planning of meetings
- The format and content of documents to be submitted and their intended dates of submission
- The design of preclinical and clinical studies and changes to preclinical or clinical protocols
- Chemistry and manufacturing issues
- Adverse events (expected and unexpected) that occur during preclinical or clinical studies

- Labeling issues and international issues (e.g., permits, inspections of foreign sites, foreign regulatory actions)
- Other topics specific to the studies or products under discussion

Preparing documents for regulatory submission is probably one of the most widely known functions of an industry regulatory group. Classic pictures of regulatory affairs groups often show them surrounded by steep piles of paper that cover dozens of tables as they prepare to submit a New Drug Application (NDA), asking for permission to make a drug available as a product. In fact, this is a monumental task (pictures don't lie), but it typically is preceded by years of previous submissions and months of work. Most of the paper on the tables was probably already submitted to the government in one form or another—at least if the company was smart. Realistically, this NDA, which usually represents about a decade of work at the company, has been preceded by dozens of previous submissions, meetings, and discussions, all of which are reflected in this huge mound of paper.

The filing of an application for a waiver to initiate clinical trials is critical to initiation of the process—in the United States, this is termed an Investigational New Drug (IND) application. Testing of a new drug in humans is only legal in the United States if the IND has been filed and the testing has not been put on clinical hold by the FDA. Clinical hold means that the FDA has concerns—usually for safety reasons—about the study design, manufacturing issues, or about the preclinical work done to date. The format, content, and submission of this document are all done under the aegis of the regulatory group.

After the initial IND filing, numerous other filings to the IND take place over the following years. Some of these are part of an annual update, and others are filed separately as specific issues arise. During clinical trials, adverse events are reported to the FDA. If the adverse reactions are serious, unexpected, or more frequent than expected, the events must be filed with the FDA within 3 to 10 days of the event, depending on whether the event was fatal or life threatening. Typically, these reports cite the nature of the problem, with background information concerning the problem and/or the patient, and they contain a summary evaluation of what this problem is likely to mean in terms of the potential risk to other patients still being tested with the drug. Dealing with this problem requires quick action and coordination with the clinical group and any other groups involved (preclinical and/or manufacturing) and is essential to building and maintaining the trust the FDA has for the company and its products.

Interacting with the internal company staff is an essential and sometimes difficult part of the job. It is the responsibility of the regulatory group to prepare reports for submission to the government that contain all the information necessary under the various regulations and guidelines. The group also makes sure the data contained in these reports are accurate and verified and that key people within research and development have the necessary training to perform the tasks relevant to the drug in development. The training must be documented, complete, and up-to-date. Often, basic researchers do not take kindly to what appear to be meddling paper pushers bugging them about how to do their jobs.

The regulatory group also participates in the strategic planning for each group to help make sure that the groups operate within government guidelines and are able to provide the necessary information required at each stage of product development. Since the information required at each stage varies according to the nature and scope of the preclinical and clinical studies to be done, it also varies according to the particular government that will review the data. Because requirements change over time, this can be a case of shooting at a moving target. This means that the negotiations required in a company to extract the necessary information and cooperation from people not in tune with government regulations during the product development cycle can be at least as challenging as dealing with the various governments that are reviewing the documentation.

Developing tactics for efficient product development and approval that can play a key role in the overall strategic plan for a company is another facet of regulatory affairs. Will the company file in the United States, in Europe, in Japan, or in all three? Although there is a movement toward harmonization in terms of the information required in these three very different markets, this process is not complete. Attempting to meet the requirements of all three regions can increase the cost of drug development sharply. Some companies enter into partnerships for foreign markets precisely because they do not want to grapple with these issues.

Some of the issues that must be examined include the kind of data that are critical for making the claims that will allow the drug to be marketed profitably and include the minimum amount of data that must be gathered to support a successful filing. We must also ask whether these minimum data will support rapid development of the drug for other uses if the first indication falls through in the clinic. Is it more important to get on the market for one indication and then follow with supplements for other indications later, or should a broader use be claimed from the beginning? Should one go after an orphan drug indication (a situation where there are so few patients that the FDA gives 7 years of market exclusivity and special tax breaks to the developer)? Clearly, the answers to these questions can have a major financial impact on the companies. The wrong decision can delay marketing of the drug for years or can limit the market—and the profitability—of a drug.

● ●
"The wrong decision can delay marketing of the drug for years or can limit the market—and the profitability—of a drug."
● ●

Because the regulatory group is on the critical path to marketing products, this group is key to a company's success. Although a company may have the brightest and best research scientists in the world working for it, unless it can bring to market the fruits of that research, the income stream for the company will be severely limited, and investors will become very unhappy.

WHAT JOBS ARE AVAILABLE IN REGULATORY AFFAIRS?

The jobs available in a regulatory group depend on the organizational scheme for the group. This varies over time within a given company (and within the government), but in general there are five different kinds of responsibilities in a regulatory group: (i) chemistry, (ii) manufacturing and controls, (iii) preclinical, (iv) clinical, and (v) compliance and documentation. In some cases, one or more of these groups is autonomous but has its own liaison person(s) to the regulatory group. In other cases, regulatory has specialists in each area who report directly to regulatory while communicating with the respective group in research and development. These jobs, which are halfway between the research and development groups on the one hand and regulatory affairs on the other, are obvious transition zones where a scientist within a company is most likely to be able to switch from a classical science job to a position in regulatory.

The chemistry, manufacturing, and control groups are responsible for documenting how the product and its raw materials are made and tested and how the manufacturing processes are controlled. In the case of companies that work primarily with small molecules, these are people with experience in synthetic chemistry and classical analytical chemistry techniques. In the case of biotechnology products, these may be molecular biologists and protein chemists. Analytical chemists and biochemists, as well as microbiologists (for sterile products), also have critical roles in this group.

Proving that a company's manufacturing methods are not only controlled but are also reproducible is a major issue with the government, which requires that these processes be validated. Validation is a series of formal tests undertaken to prove that each important step in the process can be repeated with predictable results. Even if the process undergoes changes, it is important to show that the resulting product is identical. This means that all of the equipment that must operate within very specific temperature and pressure ranges has been appropriately tested and recalibrated as needed, that the software controlling critical steps has been demonstrated to run reliably on the equipment it controls, and that changes to the software can only happen under specific and well-controlled circumstances.

The output from each person performing these tasks needs to be reported and documented to meet government requirements. When a product is to be produced commercially, the government inspects all documents to ensure that they prove the process and product are capable of reproducibly meeting the product specifications during the storage conditions specified in the marketing application. Some of these jobs fall within the regulatory world of compliance (Did people do what they said they had to do to make the product?), and some fall within the realm of documentation (Do we have all of the right reports containing the right information in the right format for the market in which we plan to sell our product?).

Preclinical Development

Preclinical development does the work needed to get the product into humans in the first place, and it provides supporting data showing that the product can reasonably be expected to be safe even if a larger population than the number of subjects in the definitive clinical trials is exposed to the product. Typically, this group studies the pharmacology and pharmacokinetics (absorption, distribution, metabolism, and excretion) of the product in various animal species, and it provides toxicology data in various species. The amount and types of animal testing required for a drug is the subject of ongoing discussions between the United States, the European Union, and Japan, and it is one area where harmonization of requirements reduced the amount of redundant testing previously performed at various stages of the drug development process.

For the preclinical group, regulatory input on the progress of the harmonization process and on the specific requirements for products in each therapeutic area is extremely important. This group also generates reports that must meet specific government requirements for content. These requirements must be taken into account when preclinical studies are designed; otherwise, more studies will have to be conducted to provide the necessary information for the IND filing. Typically, the regulatory staff and the compliance group within regulatory work hand-in-hand at each stage of the process for key studies to make sure that the study and the final report meet government requirements.

Clinical Development

The clinical group oversees the clinical trials for a product. Depending on the organization of the company and the regulatory group, this group may report to regulatory affairs, or regulatory affairs may report to them. This is another key group that is capable of making or breaking the entire company. More money is spent by this group than by any other group in the entire company, and it is their work that decides the fate of a product.

As with the preclinical group, the work of the clinical group is highly dependent on a series of regulations designed to protect the test subjects. The regulations that define this work are subject to harmonization between the different governments, but the reality is that most countries prefer to have testing done on their own particular population group before they will approve the local marketing of a new product. This can lead to a flurry of regulatory activities due to the regulations that control shipping the product for testing across international boundaries and shipping patient samples back to the company for analysis.

The government is keenly interested in each step of the clinical trial process, including the development of the protocols; enrollment of the clinical testing sites; development of the data reporting forms; verification of adherence by clinicians and nurses to the protocol; and data reporting, data entry, and adverse event reporting. Each step is subject to government inspection, and thus each is intimately involved with regulatory affairs.

Statistics, Compliance, and Documentation

Once the data are locked into the database and data verification is complete, the statisticians take over. This group grinds the data into various analyses, looking for not only the overall results, but also results by sex, race (genetic background can influence the pharmacokinetics and therefore the safety and efficacy of a drug), and population subgroup. This analysis is again subject to review by the regulatory group, as is the final report generated from each clinical trial.

The compliance group is responsible for making sure that the preclinical and clinical studies were performed as specified by a protocol that was written to meet government requirements. Depending on the organization of the company involved, they also review the chemistry, manufacturing, and control groups to ensure that their protocols, data, and reports reflect written procedures to accurately report the results of the various studies performed.

Documentation is the most obvious of all of the regulatory responsibilities. It can be the most time-consuming, tedious, and exacting of those jobs as well. People involved in this work assemble format, file, and store for instant retrieval all of the documents needed by the government to support the various filings required for a product. While this part of regulatory can be dismissed by the uninitiated as rote and as not requiring much skill, it is also true that documentation specialists put together the document that ultimately decides the fate of the product. If the reports are lost or unreadable, if the pagination and indices are mixed up or inaccurate, a decade's work can be put aside by the government until the company provides a document that is complete, comprehensible, and able to be reviewed.

For each of these areas, depending on the size of the company, at least one person is responsible for each task. In some companies, there are dozens of people responsible for each of these areas. Other companies use contract organizations to provide most of the staff and have only a few inside personnel to make sure that the functions are performed as needed.

How to Succeed in Regulatory Affairs

The specific degree and area of specialty you bring to a regulatory affairs career will determine certain aspects of your career path, although almost any area related to science can fit into this world. Animal science majors, biochemists, clinicians, chemists, ecologists, entomologists, protein chemists, molecular biologists, pharmacokineticists, plant pathologists, statisticians, veterinarians, and virologists are just some examples of the kinds of scientists who find careers in regulatory affairs.

Clearly, entomologists are more likely to find work in the Environmental Protection Agency (EPA) or with a pesticide company than in a company that makes heart valves; protein chemists are more likely to find a job in a biotech company or with the FDA than in a company that manufactures parenteral nutrient solutions. Although an advanced degree is less important in regulatory affairs than it is in academia or in basic research in industry, veterinarians are more likely to be put in charge of running large field trials of a new antibiotic for cattle than is someone with a bachelor's degree; senior management positions are more typically filled by people with advanced degrees. Exceptions to these rules abound, of course, because demonstrated ability to get the job done is extremely important in this field.

So how do you know whether this would be a good career choice for you? The first thing you need to know is which regulations govern your product area. In addition, most people find that good people skills are important, and organizational skills and the ability to store and track information are usually critical.

An ability to see the broad view without getting lost in the details is another important skill, particularly for people aiming for more senior-level management positions. A thick skin can also be an asset, particularly when acting as the bearer of bad news to top management. ("Yes, the FDA really will require us to do another $20 million clinical trial. No, the FDA won't let us claim our product cures everything in our labeling unless we prove it.")

Flexibility, the ability to change directions quickly as new information comes in, and the willingness to give up cherished plans and theories are all strong assets in this career. You may think that you know what patient group will respond best to a new drug, only to find out as the trials proceed that the drug doesn't work at all well with those patients—but it does work spectacularly well for treating another disease. You may find yourself having to deal with last-minute manufacturing changes, trying to decide what else is going to change as a result. The regulations can change, meaning that a submission that was almost ready to go out the door suddenly needs to be reorganized, or additional studies must be done. The company submitting the drug could also come up with new and inexplicable results (good or bad) with implications that have to be determined quickly: Do we stop ongoing clinical trials? Do we change trial design?

People skills are very useful in this kind of job. Product development— whether of a device, a drug, or a pesticide—requires the combined input of whole teams of specialties. As a regulatory affairs professional, it is your job to gather information from across groups and to help make sure that the story you are trying to sell to the government (or to industry) is complete and consistent. In some cases, this may mean coaxing a report in the appropriate format out of an unwilling investigator or negotiating product specifications that meet manufacturing realities, clinical necessities, and legal requirements. You can find yourself in a hostile situation when different groups in your company or agency are fighting turf wars, but you are responsible as liaison to the outside world for making all seem calm and untroubled. You could also be the one who helps to get new laws passed to protect consumers, acting for your consumer group in a position where your ability to get the job done depends primarily on your powers of persuasion.

The ability to hear accurately not only what people are saying but also what they are *not* saying can be crucial. In working for the government, you may find yourself in a position in which, because of your experience with similar products, you expect that a product may have effects clearly unanticipated by the manufacturer. In this case, you must get the company to do the necessary evaluations—but you may not be able to tell it why because the explanation would give them confidential information about a potentially competing product in development. These hints can be essential for getting your product to the market quickly, and you need to know when to push for more information and when to quit while you are ahead.

Keeping Things Organized

Organizational skills are very important as well. The typical NDA can be 200 volumes of more than 400 pages each, reflecting data acquired over 10 or more years of research. Organizing that information as it comes in, sorting it, storing it, and assembling it is a monumental job, requiring whole teams of people working for months. On the government end, reading and absorbing the information, quickly finding key questions, and coordinating the overall response to the company in the short timetable dictated under the new user's fees rules can be tough. But when you realize that most companies are working against management goals of "x number of NDAs filed per year," you can imagine that the Christmas rush has a whole new meaning to the receiving docks in Washington. Keeping track of the various documents you are supposed to review, of what company responded to which query (and which issues are still outstanding), and preparing thoughtful written reviews of each application on time puts demands on anyone's filing system.

More and more, a talent for strategic planning is becoming essential as regulatory professionals are asked to assist in overall product development planning. Taking into account existing and in-process regulations and guidelines can help determine the probable development times and risks for a new product. The ability to successfully predict the quickest and most likely pathways to the marketing of a product has been known to make or break a young start-up company that has only limited financial resources available to stay alive long enough to get a product to market.

• •
"More and more, a talent for strategic planning is becoming essential as regulatory professionals are asked to assist in overall product development planning."
• •

Being in regulatory affairs has its downsides, too, as with any other job. An additional useful job skill is to be able to deal with the sequelae of being the bearer of bad tidings. Because regulatory professionals are the interface with the government, for some people within a company, they are viewed almost as being part of the government. Regulations passed to prevent problems caused by other companies sometimes seem to become the fault of the regulatory affairs group. Similarly, reports of compliance problems spotted by the company's own regulatory group can be greeted with ingratitude. The regulatory group frequently shares the blame when the government refuses to permit the marketing of a new product.

Never forget that over the years, you develop a reputation within your area. If you have the reputation for straight shooting and fair evaluation based on good science and backed by the facts, you are more likely to get things done in your own organization and with the companies or government agencies with which you deal.

HOW DO YOU GET INTO REGULATORY AFFAIRS?

If you ask 100 people in this field how they got their current job, you will probably get at least 75 different answers. The answer depends a lot on whether you want to work for government, industry, or consumer groups. Most people have the common denominator of some form of science background. But lawyers, those with M.B.A.s, and the occasional mathematician have been known to sneak in as well. It is common for a person to start as a scientist in government and switch over to industry because the "on-the-job" training in working with regulators is often highly prized by industry. While government jobs tend to be fairly low-paying, the initial investment in time spent training can pay off if you do decide to move to an industrial job or to strike out on your own as a regulatory consultant. Jobs in the consumer industry are less visible, and there are fewer of them.

Most commonly, scientists move into regulatory affairs as part of a career evolution. As a scientist, you can run into glass ceilings—jobs where no further promotion is likely. In some cases, career progression is blocked by the lack of an advanced degree. In other cases, your scientific specialty is simply not likely to lead to a high-level management opportunity. For example, few toxicologists ever become officers of a company unless they leave their own narrow specialty.

Other people find that they prefer dealing with the wider spectrum of information—they find molecular biology too specialized, too out of touch with everyday reality. And for some, finding a science-related job that gets them out of the lab is a strong attraction. Biologists can develop allergies to the animals they work with, and they may start looking for some way to use their knowledge away from the bench. Don't count on a 9:00-to-5:00 job, however, particularly if you work for a small and growing company.

One way to move into government is to get a post-doctoral fellowship or the equivalent, working at the FDA, the Centers for Disease Control (CDC), or the EPA. There are various entry-level jobs in the government testing labs that can migrate to the divisions of the government that review marketing applications or that perform inspections. Jobs in the FDA are listed on its Web site and are also listed in *Science* or in other scientific journals. People in the military may be able to transfer to the Public Health Service, which staffs various positions within the FDA and the CDC. Carl Peck, a physician in the military who was very interested in pharmacokinetics, went this route and eventually became the Director of the Center for Drug Evaluation and Research at the FDA. This also can be a popular route for people who have had their advanced degrees paid for by the government and who owe the government service time as payback. The National Institutes of Health (NIH) is also a breeding ground for government regulators-to-be because various clinical trials are conducted by NIH, and there is extensive contact between the FDA, CDC, and NIH.

In industry, there are also many routes. One common route is to start out in the lab, gathering data and writing reports for submission to a regulatory agency, learning in the process about the regulations affecting your area, and then moving over into regulatory when a job opens up. Another route is to find an entry-level position as one of the people responsible for assembling and tracking the mounds of paper that are required to support products, then gradually becoming responsible for more strategic decisions on larger projects.

In companies that have project management groups (usually larger companies), scientists sometimes move over to these groups first, learning the wider scope of product development, before finally ending up in regulatory. In a small company, this result can be reached by a much less logical route—the company needs to have something done, you are bright and available, so you are elected to get it done!

In general, the potential for switching around between jobs and developing titles and responsibilities that reflect your skills are greater in smaller companies, but larger companies provide more jobs and opportunities for getting a toe in the door. Logically enough, even small companies prefer to hire someone with a wealth of previous experience.

CROs as Starting Points

You can also start by getting a job with a contract research organization. These companies provide contract services to the pharmaceutical industry by doing various parts of the product development process such as preclinical testing, analytical work, manufacturing, statistical evaluation, and clinical trials. Many of these companies have entry-level positions available. To find these companies, look on the Internet or look at lists organized by the various regulatory societies. One such list is entitled *Pharmaceutical Contract Support Organizations,* which is issued by the Drug Information Association (DIA). Once you have some training as a scientist who is responsible for generating data that are reviewed by the government, you can move over into regulatory affairs as a veteran who has survived (successfully) regulatory inspections and dealing with the government.

There are many courses and training seminars available where you can learn the regulations. There are courses and seminars offered by societies involved with regulatory affairs, such as the DIA, Regulatory Affairs Professionals (RAPs), and the Food and Drug Law Institute. Each of these groups has a Web page that lists upcoming seminars. You can also join these societies and get on their mailing lists—you can even join some of them online.

It is also true, however, that neither course work and seminars nor academic training can provide real-world experience. The diversity of scientific specialties in regulatory affairs reflects the simple fact that this is a career that requires on-the-job training. The best experience is gained through dealing

"The diversity of scientific specialties in regulatory affairs reflects the simple fact that this is a career that requires on-the-job training."

with information that is typically highly confidential to a company; this limits the value of generalized seminars.

It is also important to get to know the people and personalities on the other end of the phone line when dealing with tough issues. No regulations can—or should—be extensive enough to fit all cases. Most decisions are made on the basis of what has worked successfully under reasonably similar situations. The dream product that nicely and tamely fits itself into the published regulations is a rare bird. Creativity in interpreting and applying the rules and guidelines is often required when new areas of research begin to give rise to new modalities of therapy, such as gene therapy.

Regulatory affairs professionals occupy jobs at almost all levels within government and industry, from data entry personnel to the commissioner of the FDA. In industry, they rarely become chief executive officers or presidents, but they may be senior vice presidents or executive vice presidents of regulatory affairs. As stated earlier, it is common for people to choose this career simply to avoid glass ceilings. But if your aim is to become a corporate mogul, amassing billions and billions in personal fortune, regulatory affairs is probably not the best career choice. Regulatory affairs can, however, become a satisfying and rewarding profession.

One nice aspect true of this profession is that once you have gained a reputation for knowledge and professionalism in your field, you can strike out on your own as a consultant. This is intriguing for entrepreneurial types who like to boldly forge ahead on their own, marketing themselves and their skills to companies that do not really want to set up permanently the staff needed to bring a product to market. Sometimes consultants are also hired to bring in experience for a type of product that is new to the company or to help a company with strategic planning.

The government sometimes brings in consultants to help solve a specific science question. Consultants roam from project to project, and Nancy Chew, a regulatory consultant for many years, has described regulatory consulting as being done best by someone who is easily bored. The nature of the job changes from project to project. It is not, however, for someone who is just starting out in the industry because having a track record of success is critical in your marketing.

In summary, a career in regulatory affairs can be stimulating and challenging, and it can make extensive use of your scientific training. It requires in-depth knowledge and a tactical view of the regulations and the product, diplomatic skills, and a willingness to dive into details without becoming overwhelmed by them. But most of all, it requires a clear mind that is able to tie together all the scientific disciplines needed to make a product.

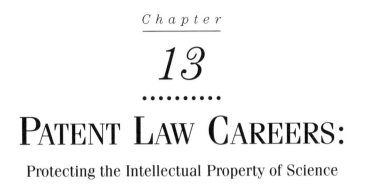

Chapter

13

••••••••••

PATENT LAW CAREERS:

Protecting the Intellectual Property of Science

•••••••••••••••••

Alexandra J. Baran, Ph.D.

President, A.J. Baran Consulting, Inc.

When I graduated from Stanford University in 1982 with my Ph.D. in organic chemistry, the last place I expected my career to lead was the law. I had watched my (now ex-) husband suffer through courses at a prominent law school to reach his goal of becoming a corporate attorney in a major law firm. In college, I had taken exactly one political science course to fulfill a distribution requirement and had secretly disdained my friends who seemed to sell their souls to get into law school. I thought I had no aptitude for legal reasoning—nor did I want any. Now, 20-something years later, I have been practicing patent law as an agent for 11 years and would never go back to the lab.

PATENTS AND PRACTITIONERS

A patent is a legal instrument granting the owner the right to make, use, or sell an invention and to exclude others from doing so. In the United States, an inventor is entitled to a patent if an invention is novel, useful, and unobvious. Patents in foreign countries can be obtained on a similar basis.

Patents are vitally important in areas of commerce where a strong patent ensures the profitability of a product. Patent practitioners are concerned with patent prosecution (the activities associated with obtaining a patent from a nation's patent office), as differentiated from patent litigation (enforcing a patent in court in the context of a lawsuit). Other related activities include license negotiation (in which the patent owner lets others use the invention for a price), portfolio management (strategies for surrounding a basic patent with related patents), portfolio analysis, legal opinion work, and litigation support.

The term *patent practitioner* encompasses both patent attorneys and patent agents. All practitioners must pass a federal bar exam administered by the U.S. Patent and Trademark Office (PTO) before being permitted to represent clients in their quest to obtain patents. Agents must have appropriate scientific qualifications; attorneys must have a law degree *and* the appropriate scientific qualifications. Attorneys also must pass the bar exam of the state in which they wish to practice law. As a practical matter, it makes no difference to the PTO whether you are an agent or an attorney. However, agents are restricted from the general practice of law and cannot represent a client in a conventional courtroom.

Like attorneys, registered patent agents are legal professionals and are required to adhere to strict standards of professional conduct and canons of ethics. These canons are the same as those set forth by the American Bar Association for attorneys. These rules cover things like dishonesty, fraud, deceit, misrepresentation, mishandling of client funds, and, my personal favorite, moral turpitude. You can lose your registration to practice, and thus your livelihood, if you are found to violate these rules. If such compliance bothers you, you should *not* consider a career in law.

My (Convoluted) Career Path

I attribute my childhood interest in science to my parents even though they were not highly educated, nor scientists by trade. My father encouraged my mathematical and mechanical abilities in ways such as teaching me how to test the vacuum tubes in our television. My college physics teacher later marveled at the fact that I knew how to splice electrical wires, a skill that today is still far too uncommon in young women. My mother's own interest in plants and animals encouraged me to observe the natural world in fine detail. When I was in high school, she pushed me to become a volunteer at the local hospital so that I might develop an interest in medicine. At the same time, my high school English and French teachers encouraged me to develop my language skills.

When I chose a college, I knew I wanted to double major in English and a science. I graduated from Mount Holyoke College with an A.B. degree in chemistry and English. Because I wanted to make certain that I could support myself, I chose chemistry over English literature for graduate school and entered Stanford University. I joined the research group of Professor Harry S. Mosher, a well-known stereochemist. Harry had earlier discovered the chemical structure of the natural product tetrodotoxin, the stuff that gives puffer fish their buzz.

• •

"Because I wanted to make certain that I could support myself, I chose chemistry over English literature for graduate school and entered Stanford University."

• •

During my fourth year at Stanford, I realized that I wasn't cut out for laboratory research. I found bench work lonely, isolating, and frustratingly slow. I was reasonably good at it, being meticulous and detail-oriented. The parts of my graduate career in which I excelled were research planning and oral presentations. Because Stanford was in the business of training professors, we were required to write two novel research proposals and give two public seminars ("chalk talks" without slides) long before our dissertation defenses and oral exams. I ascribe my success in these endeavors to the written and oral communication skills I honed at Mt. Holyoke analyzing Chaucer with Carolyn P. Collette and *Bleak House* with Jean Sundrann.

My suspicions from graduate school were confirmed during my first job as a bench chemist in discovery research at Stauffer Chemical Company, designing and making insecticides. I could think of compounds much faster than I could synthesize them myself. In spite of my early success at the bench (I was named inventor on five patents), Stauffer was not going to give a brand-new chemist a research group to run. The clincher came when I sought treatment for my lifelong allergies and my doctor said to me: "Why on earth are you a chemist? Get your body out of the lab as soon as possible!" For a supposedly intelligent person, it had never occurred to me that someone with every allergy known to man should not be a chemist.

At first, I decided to move into research management as soon as possible. Stauffer obliged by allowing me to take some management courses. My goal was temporarily interrupted by a move to Texas (the now ex-husband's idea) and a 3-year stint as a research chemist at Pennzoil Products Company. Although I was again successful (two more patents and a commercial product), I decided that I did not go to Stanford to pour one gooey liquid into another gooey liquid and thus sought an escape.

In 1984, two professors, a neurobiologist and an ophthalmologist, founded Houston Biotechnology Incorporated (HBI) with patented technology licensed from Baylor College of Medicine. The immunotoxin (ricin A chain linked to a monoclonal antibody specific to lens epithelial cells) was designed to prevent secondary cataract, a common complication of primary cataract surgery. In addition, the company had also licensed from Texas A&M University a patent covering use of a small organic molecule to treat glaucoma. Manufacturing this small molecule required knowledge of stereoselective organic synthesis, which happened to be my dissertation topic. A recruiter introduced me to the company in 1986, and I became its eighth employee. My job was to set up and manage an organic lab sufficient to synthesize the small molecule and similar compounds. I had reached my goal of research management, or so I thought.

About 3 months after I joined HBI, we received a letter from an obscure pharmaceutical company named Merck inviting us to review one of their patents. To make a long and ridiculous story short, I suddenly had no molecule to synthesize. At the same time, the correspondence concerning the patents HBI had licensed from Baylor had formed a foot-high pile on the neurobiologist cofounder's desk. He turned to me and said, "Here. You're an inventor, right? You understand these. *Do* something with them."

During the next 7½ years, I managed our rapidly growing portfolio of licensed and self-generated patents, using outside patent counsel to handle the direct prosecution. I also acquired numerous other responsibilities, as is common in start-up companies, and was made a vice president shortly before HBI went public.

HBI had achieved early notoriety in financial circles by raising $23.8 million in a limited research partnership public offering a month after the October 1987 stock market crash. The downside was that financing structure made the eventual public stock offering difficult to achieve and not very profitable. In addition, I became extremely uncomfortable with the direction the company was heading from a scientific and management perspective.

That discomfort, combined with my fervent desire to leave Texas, caused me to reevaluate my career options. (And, yes, my ex is still in Texas.) I considered some of the other career paths mentioned in this book, including business development, and investment banking. I interviewed for business development positions at other start-up companies but kept remembering that several of HBI's outside patent lawyers had tried to recruit me over the years to join their firms.

Eventually, I said yes to one of those firms. They moved me back to California, paid for my patent bar review course, and would have sent me to law school part-time had I so desired. Unfortunately for that firm, 6 months later, the partner I was working with and I were recruited to start the new Silicon Valley biotech patent practice at Weil, Gotshal, & Manges, LLP. My career at Weil was successful, and I developed my own client base.

One of my clients was SunPharm Pharmaceutical Company, a start-up founded by Stefan Borg with technology licensed from the University of Florida. (Mr. Borg was involved in Houston Biotechnology and the same brave soul who taught business development to Dr. Robbins-Roth, as described in her chapter in this book. Stefan was the most honorable business person I have ever known.) After another year, Dr. Rich Neeley, a well-known biotech patent attorney, recruited me to join Cooley Godward, LLP. I was quite pleased to join Cooley, a powerhouse high-tech firm, which had been Houston Biotechnology's corporate and patent law firm during much of my tenure at HBI.

Although SunPharm came with me to Cooley as a patent prosecution client, my practice evolved to include a high percentage of intellectual property portfolio evaluation work for investment banking and venture capital clients. The strength of, and the potential risks associated with, a company's patents contributes heavily to a bank's willingness to underwrite a public or private offering and to an investor's willingness to invest. Such risk assessment is more typically done by patent attorneys as opposed to agents, but my previous experience with raising capital at HBI made it possible for me to keep my clients very happy with my analyses. (I often said, "Do *not* invest.") When I left Cooley, my practice consisted of one-third direct patent prosecution, one-third patent portfolio management, and one-third analysis work.

My departure from Cooley was not voluntary. In August 1991, Cooley let go 15% of its legal professionals, in the midst of a 2-year wave of layoffs from Silicon Valley law firms. (Laying off lawyers is a bad idea; some of the firms that did so no longer exist or have suffered permanently bruised reputations.) Before my severance pay ran out, I joined a local public biotech company as associate director, patent administration, reporting to the general counsel.

• • • • • • • • • • • • • • • • • • • •
"I left as soon as I could to start my own solo practice."
• • • • • • • • • • • • • • • • • • • •

When that position turned out to be considerably less than advertised and my stock options tanked 3 months later, I left as soon as I could to start my own solo practice. I had always wanted to try this option and still had enough contacts from my time at Cooley to make it viable. My current practice is styled as a "consulting firm" because I am not an attorney, and thus, "not a professional" according to the corporate laws of California. I am now happy as a clam, or rather, a fish. (My royal blue beta Boris keeps me good company in my office.)

A TYPICAL DAY

If you are a patent practitioner whose practice comprises mostly direct patent prosecution, a typical day is spent writing applications and preparing responses to PTO examiners. Depending on the technology involved, an application can take 10 to 50 hours to prepare. Most of this time is spent in solitary review of related technology (prior art). You then turn the written scientific description and data obtained from the inventor(s) into appropriate patent "legalese." Although this process is lonely and requires intense concentration, it is also highly creative and is the aspect of prosecution I enjoy the most.

After a patent application is filed, the prosecution phase begins in earnest. A patent examiner writes an "office action" in which he or she tells you that the invention in question is already known, worthless, and obvious to any qualified scientist with half a brain. You respond, in writing and very politely, saying that the invention is truly the best thing since sliced bread and that, if the examiner would simply read the prior art correctly, he would recognize your inventor's true creativity. Responding to patent office examiners requires a different kind of creativity on the practitioner's part because you must synthesize good legal argument with good science and then write a response following the arcane and precise formats of the patent office.

Social contact can be quite variable. Some days, the phone can ring off the hook with panicked clients. Other days, it is just you and the e-mails. Face-to-face meetings with inventors can be very stimulating and productive but generally occur only at the very beginning of the patenting process. Interaction with colleagues also varies depending on whether you work at a law firm or in another environment. In

● ●

"Face-to-face meetings with inventors can be very stimulating and productive but generally occur only at the very beginning of the patenting process."

● ●

law firms, the dreaded "billable hour" rules. Attorneys and agents must "bill" (charge for time actually worked) a certain number of hours per year, typically between 1700 to 2200 hours depending the particular firm. Your total compensation often is directly tied to hours billed. Billable time does not include necessary tasks such as keeping up with the scientific literature and the constant changes in the patent rules and law. If you are on the partnership track, you are also expected to manage staff and to develop new clients. Thus, since you are constantly worried about fulfilling your billable quota, you tend to limit your interaction with your firm colleagues during the day. In corporations, time pressures still exist, but the emphasis is on getting the job done instead of the time a task takes to accomplish. Please note that salaries at firms do tend to be higher than those in corporations and other institutions.

ATTORNEY VERSUS AGENT

Anyone who has already spent years in graduate school obtaining a master's degree or a doctorate in science or engineering may well cringe at the idea of going back to school for a law degree. The cringing increases exponentially with the number of years in the workforce after graduate school.

Moving into patent law mid-career is not that unusual. A friend of mine from graduate school spent 20 years as a highly successful research chemist at a major chemical company (scores of patents and numerous commercial products) until the company decided to close his business unit. Fortunately, the company offered him the opportunity to move into the law department, where they trained him in patent prosecution. He now enjoys his work as a patent agent. His story is typical of agents in large corporations, where scientists with good writing skills are recruited from the bench and trained. The possibility of attending law school part-time and on the company's nickel is also available.

• •

"The possibility of attending law school part-time and on the company's nickel is also available."

• •

If you are considering moving to patent law directly from graduate school or a post-doctoral position, the question of whether to get a J.D. becomes more problematic. In the long run, you can make more money with the J.D. because of the possibility of becoming a partner in a law firm. If you don't get a law degree and become a patent agent instead, you will still make more money as a patent practitioner than as a bench scientist with comparable years of experience.

As for going to law school, the drill is the same as if you entered directly from college: take the LSAT, apply, get in, and go full-time (3 years) or part-time (generally 4 to 5 years). In my case, the unnerving experience of sitting in a Rice University classroom to take the heavily proctored LSAT surrounded by kids young enough to be my own children was proof enough that I could not tolerate sitting in a law classroom for 3 to 5 years.

My personal decision not to obtain a J.D. was also heavily influenced by the fact that I already had had a successful career in the biotech industry, where I had made many contacts whom then translated into clients once I joined a law firm. I should emphasize that my ability to develop my own client base so quickly is very unusual for an agent. In law firms, patent agents generally get their work assignments and clients from a supervising attorney. Junior attorneys find themselves in a similar situation but are expected to develop clients as they move along the track to partnership. More senior agents may be able to develop a personal client base, but an attorney at the firm will always supervise them.

This last fact points out a downside of being a patent practitioner if you do not become an attorney: you cannot become a partner in a U.S. law firm, which substantially limits your income potential. (In Canada, patent agents can become partners in intellectual property law firms.) For agents, who in many cases have more academic education and life experience than patent attorneys with 3-year law degrees and a few undergraduate science courses, this point can be quite frustrating.

On the other hand, partnership in a law firm also has its drawbacks, including real monetary exposure if the firm experiences financial difficulties. Opportunities for advancement in corporations are also limited for agents in that they cannot fill certain positions such as general counsel. However, with the right skills and ambition, you may be able to advance into other positions.

Necessary Skills and Personality Traits

• •
"Many of the skills that enabled you to get a graduate degree in science or engineering translate well into the skills necessary for the successful practice of law."
• •

Many of the skills that enabled you to get a graduate degree in science or engineering translate well into the skills necessary for the successful practice of law. Analytical abilities including logical thought, pattern recognition, and classification ability; organizational skills are also important. Careful attention to detail is very valuable. The direct technical expertise you obtained in your field of specialization, whether it was a detailed knowledge of chemical synthesis, gene splicing, or computer programming, becomes less important than your ability to learn new science in your art area by asking insightful questions of your client inventors. Your already proven ability to learn science is just as important as the science you have already learned.

On the other hand, legal reasoning is not intuitive to all scientists. The law is based on concepts, not concrete physical data, and it is constantly evolving. Legal opinions are just that: opinions formed from a detailed analysis of apparent facts with a good deal of judgment thrown in. Such analyses are abstract and rely on the interpretation of the very arcane historical practice of patent law. You must be comfortable with ambiguity and be satisfied by logical argument to enjoy this profession.

Other talents not common to all scientists are good communication and interpersonal skills. You must be able to communicate clearly and concisely, both in written and oral form. Good English grammar and diction are required; foreign language skills are a plus. Often, entire days will be spent reading and writing, so it is helpful if you like these activities. Oral skills become important in two ways: client communication and client education. A truly effective patent practitioner is able to tease important details from a sometimes-reluctant inventor. Further, the more the inventor understands patent law, the more likely he or she is to be cooperative. Thus, teaching skills are important.

You must realize that law is fundamentally a service profession. Your ability to keep your clients happy is crucial to your success. You are no longer allowed to be an eccentric scientist yourself; peculiar scientists are now your valuable clients and must often be coddled. In addition, your real clients, representatives of the entities that own the inventor's patents, must also be treated well. Finally, knowing how to deal with opposing counsel (lawyers representing clients adverse to your own) with courtesy goes a long way toward your client's success.

JOB RESOURCES

The first resource you should explore is the user-friendly Web site of the U.S. Patent & Trademark Office (www.uspto.gov). The site gives an introduction to the patenting process, provides definitions for terms like *invention*, and, most importantly, posts the "General Requirements Bulletin for Admission to the Examination to Practice in Patent Cases Before the U.S. PTO." This bulletin delineates the scientific course work required for eligibility to sit for the patent bar. The PTO is rather fussy about these requirements, but you might as well get used to it, since patent law is a picky business.

Now that you have determined you are interested and qualified, how do you find a job as a patent practitioner? If you have decided to take the law school route directly after science or engineering graduate school, you will naturally fall into the law firm recruiting cycle on campus. If you have decided to become an agent and have not been recruited to do so by your existing employer, there are law firms that hire scientists and engineers as technical assistants and then support their training as agents. Such positions generally include the option of the firm financing law school on a part-time basis in exchange for a specified commitment to the firm.

Several good hard copy and online resources exist for locating these programs. Martindale Hubbell is the granddaddy of all legal compendia and is now available on the Internet (www.martindale.com) with links to the Web sites of individual intellectual property law firms. The American Intellectual Property Lawyers Association (www.aipla.org) also gives links to members. Many law firms post articles about intellectual property on their Web sites and also provide links to other useful patent sites.

Another useful resource is the National Association for Law Placement (NALP), the organization that keeps law schools, law firms, and other legal employers honest in their recruitment and hiring practices. A particularly useful feature of the NALP Web site (www.NALP.org) is the annual salary survey information. Base salaries for associate attorneys at law firms vary depending on years of experience and on the size of the firm. In 2002, they ranged from $60,000 to $165,000 according to NALP. In general, patent lawyers receive a salary premium, especially if they hold doctorates. Salaries for patent partners vary according to seniority and their own "book" of business.

Patent agents command a similarly wide range of salaries, but exact information is difficult to obtain. As with any profession, compensation for patent practitioners is negotiable at law firms and in industry. Base salaries may be fixed in a lock-step fashion, especially at large firms. However, bonuses, stock options, and other forms of compensation offer additional flexibility.

New agents and attorneys should realize that the first several years on the job are an apprenticeship; considerable time and effort on the part of more senior practitioners will be devoted to making you a valuable contributor. The first milestone comes with passing the patent bar, which typically occurs in the first year or so. Approximately 3 to 5 years of training are necessary before you are qualified to take on your own clients. When you do enable that first client to get a patent issued, however, you will find it just as exciting as if you were the inventor yourself.

14

• • • • • • • • • •

ENTERING BIOMEDICAL
AND SCIENTIFIC CONSULTING

• • • • • • • • • • • • • • • •

Robert Roth, M.D., Ph.D.
Medical Director, THE WEINBERG GROUP, INC.

For the past 5-plus years, I have been medical director of a Washington, D.C.-based scientific consulting company with several satellite offices, including one in San Francisco. For me, this was a middle-age career change from an academic comfort zone I'd known for quite a long time to an occupation with a whole new set of challenges. Looking back, I'm glad to have had two distinct careers rather than just one. I think many of us in science can be productive and satisfied in a range of occupations, and switching fields is not so bad once inertia has been overcome.

• •
"I think many of us in science can be productive and satisfied in a range of occupations, and switching fields is not so bad once inertia has been overcome."
• •

LEAVING THE COMFORT ZONE OF ACADEMIA

My transition to an alternative career in science began after many years in academia. I had been an assistant professor at the University of California with a medical degree and Ph.D. in biochemistry. In the typical career of the clinician–scientist at an academic medical center, this meant combining research, teaching, and service work. While my research was stimulating, the clinical work was generally routine, and the nasty hospital politics were, unfortunately, also generally routine. I was wasting a considerable fraction of my time writing grants that wouldn't get funded. I had become very specialized scientifically, a true expert in only a couple of narrow clinical fields. As is typical in academia, my service work and teaching were in subjects that I knew well, and I wasn't really learning much new. Although I didn't fully realize it until after I entered the consulting world, in my day-to-day life at the university I was using only a very small fraction of my biochemistry and medical knowledge and experience.

As federal funding for research gradually began to disappear, I realized I would have to change from a research focus to more of an administrative one if I were to stay at the university. I am admittedly fairly hardheaded and obstinate, and such a shift was not at all appealing. Although I loved the basic research part of my life, the lack of appreciation for my teaching and service efforts was a constant source of frustration. So, when I finally left the university, my attitude was admittedly not the greatest. In many respects, I identified with the message of a favorite academia cartoon from the *New Yorker*: a professor's gravestone, which reads "Published, but perished anyway." I didn't know what I wanted to do next, but I was pretty sure it wasn't more of the same. Other academic opportunities in the Bay Area were few, and I really didn't want to move. So it seemed most reasonable to examine other avenues.

The Transition: Not So Difficult After All

I had contacted a number of local biotechnology companies looking for research opportunities but found no good fits with my level of expertise and experience. Clinical opportunities probably existed, but I had no background in conducting clinical trials. In addition, such a career change didn't pass the "fun" smell test. Luckily, a friend who also was an ex-academic physician knew of my in-limbo situation and convinced me to visit his consulting group and look into working with them part-time. As is so often the case, the driving force for a career choice was serendipity.

This consulting group, which I joined, was a small outfit that worked with early stage biopharmaceutical and medical device companies and the investors who funded them. I got to critique start-up business plans for investors, work through the pros and cons of development plan strategies for new health care products, and evaluate the opportunities and risks of new technologies. I rapidly discovered that these activities allowed me to use my scientific and medical knowledge to a much greater extent than during my academic (read: specialized) career. I also realized that these projects demanded that I constantly learn something new. These two features were what convinced me I had found my new direction.

About a year later, the founder of the consulting group decided to move the company elsewhere, but I was not interested in moving. This initial introduction to consulting had been so positive that I had no trouble deciding that another consulting job was at the top of my list. My job opportunity presented itself the old-fashioned way, in the newspaper want ads. An established east coast–based scientific consulting company was looking to expand its west coast office in San Francisco and in the process hopefully expand its regional profile and client base. I answered the ad and met with the CEO shortly thereafter. When I learned of the broad scope of the company's clients and projects, and the caliber of the consulting team, I was hooked.

Putting My Scientific Background to Work

My very first project in the new consulting company proved to me how extensively my scientific and medical background could serve me in the consulting world. A client had asked us to provide an overview of the clinical state of stem cell replacement therapy and to assess the competitive market environment for device products involved in processing and manipulating stem cells. To produce a very detailed report for the client, I was able to use my medical knowledge of standard and experimental stem cell therapies. My years in the research laboratory allowed me to identify a host of critical issues related to cell culture and the use of growth factors. Although the client couched the assignment as a business opportunity evaluation, what they really needed was detailed input from a scientist's perspective to identify major difficulties in the technical development of their system and to assess the state of the current science in stem cell biology; they also needed the clinician's perspective regarding the potential clinical benefit over the existing state of the art.

In the years since this first assignment, I have undertaken scores of projects in which a strong scientific base provided the level of detail required to help the client. In many instances, the ability to comprehend and critically evaluate the scientific literature provided the basis for my conclusions and recommendations. The detail orientation of my scientific training and background and the skills I developed over the years to critically and objectively evaluate data have proved useful over and over.

> "The detail orientation of my scientific training and background and the skills I developed over the years to critically and objectively evaluate data have proved useful over and over."

WHO WE ARE AND WHAT WE DO

The firm where I work, THE WEINBERG GROUP, is a scientific and regulatory consulting firm. Many of our clients are the manufacturers of health care products, consumer products, chemicals, and a host of other industries that have needs and problems based in science. Other clients who come to us because of scientific issues are law firms, national advocacy groups and associations, and investors. In broad terms, we help companies get their products to market and keep their products on the market. We focus, as much as possible, on finding science-based solutions to help clients under pressure from difficult product development problems, threatened or enacted regulatory action, legal attack, and economic risks. Solutions can range from technical analyses of published and unpublished information to experience-based advisory insights and everything in between. Although we perform many of the routine clinical and regulatory functions commonly outsourced from biomedical companies to consultants, the jobs that keep us excited are those in which the client is at great risk, and our input is instrumental in achieving a saving outcome.

The company, founded more than 20 years ago, has ranged in size over recent years between 50 and 100 people. We are organized in broad practices based on the expertise of the practice directors and the focus of the work: U.S. pharmaceuticals, clinical pharmacology and biopharmaceutics, epidemiology and biostatistics, compliance and quality management, medical devices, applied toxicology and risk sciences, U.S. science-based advocacy, European advocacy, and product defense. Although each of us fills a specific spot within the organizational chart, most of us end up working across practices to a considerable extent. We also work across practices as teams, as needed. For example, in working on a New Drug Application, we are likely to use staff from each of the first four practices listed above.

What we do is harder to define because, as I often explain to prospective clients, it is actually "all over the map." In the Federal Food and Drug Administration (FDA)-regulated health care arena, we provide support for clients' clinical, regulatory, and business development needs. In the environmental science, health and ecological risk, and toxicology arenas, we tackle risk assessment or advocacy needs, as well as contributing to regulatory policy. In an area we call product defense and litigation support, we educate lawyers, develop scientific arguments and counterarguments, and identify expert witnesses in cases of biomedical product liability. In the broad area of product stewardship, we provide analytic, technical, and strategic input for clients with a major product at risk.

Some projects are long-term support roles for a client who has "outsourced" a function to our consulting company. An example would be our activities as a drug company's outsourced drug safety and surveillance department; such projects can last years. Other complicated, time-consuming projects that we undertake as regulatory consultants include preparation of FDA documents. Such projects may require the work of a half-dozen of us or more, taking months to complete, and can ultimately generate a series of documents extensive enough to fill many boxes. For this type of project, there needs to be lots of attention to detail and considerable management effort to ensure everything gets done correctly and on time; a poorly produced document could end up costing the client millions of dollars. These types of projects can be tour de force efforts and are true team efforts.

At the other end of the spectrum from large outsourced activities are more directed projects that provide answers to a very specific scientific question or give expert advice on a specific issue. These projects, which constitute the vast majority of jobs we undertake, provide most of the variety and intellectual stimulation that make consulting fun. To give an idea of the scientific breadth of these jobs, here are examples from my own experience.

- Evaluation of a pharmaceutical start-up opportunity for an investor
- Due diligence reporting on an in-licensing drug candidate
- Assessment of whether a product's side effects constitute a true health risk and the likelihood that such problems could result in litigation
- Evaluation of whether clinical data from a drug trial fully support the sponsor's conclusions and would withstand an FDA audit
- In-depth white paper analysis on the clinical potential and technical risks of a new biomedical technology
- Literature-based critical analysis on how the epidemiology of a communicable disease has changed over the decades
- State-of-the-science review of how effective current methods are to minimize the risk of bovine spongiform encephalitis transmission from cow-derived proteins used in pharmaceuticals
- Recommendations of the best design for a clinical trial of a medical device
- Identifying and assessing the seriousness of potential risks from an unapproved experimental cancer drug that was given to patients without any prior animal or human exposure data
- Ghost writing of a paper for publication

Most of these projects demand critical thinking, creativity and judgment, and often involve considerable literature research and synthesis, much like when writing a college term paper. For projects such as these, our value and reputation as consultants derive from expertise and industry knowledge, ability to integrate information, and a focus based on objective, scientific approaches rather than opinion.

Limited only by a link to some aspect of science, we provide a wide range of client services, as described previously. I should point out here that this range of services is somewhat unusual in the scientific consulting world. Much more often, a scientific consulting firm will be more niche-based, specializing in a particular aspect of expertise such as clinical development, regulatory guidance, or environmental toxicology.

To serve this variety of functions, we have developed a professional staff with a very broad range of expertise. We have invested in the expertise of physicians with a range of backgrounds; a battery of scientists with Ph.D.s with backgrounds in all the basic and applied biomedical sciences, including epidemiology and biostatistics; ex-VPs of clinical, regulatory, research or other disciplines from major companies of the biopharmaceutical world; a biomedical product liability lawyer; and an ex-FDA senior director. Clearly, this range of skill sets allows us to contribute to a very large variety of projects. But the real beauty, from my perspective, is that our collaborative projects allow all of us to continually learn from each other and expand our own technical zones of comfort.

"But the real beauty, from my perspective, is that our collaborative projects allow all of us to continually learn from each other and expand our own technical zones of comfort."

The Company Structure

In contrast to the giant consulting companies of the world, we don't have a division of managers and a division of workers. Most of us act as active contributors on projects no matter where we fall in the company structure. At times, even the CEO may contribute to the heavy lifting of whatever analysis and report writing is required for a project. Consequently, the majority of us do billable work, with only a small number of strictly administrative employees serving nonreimbursable functions such as human resources and marketing. That said, we and most other consulting companies our size have some sort of hierarchy and billing structure based on skills, capabilities, and, to some extent, level of scientific training and professional degree.

Excluding the administrative staff, the remaining personnel constitute a diamond-shaped organizational structure. At the top, there are a limited number of practice directors, with primary responsibility to bring in business, manage projects, and provide high-level strategic consulting to clients.

Salaries of practice directors are negotiable, depending greatly on extent of consulting experience, ability to attract new clients, and other such factors. At the other end of the organizational chart are the junior researcher staff members, generally recent college graduates gaining work experience before going on to some postgraduate program. Researchers primarily perform literature searches, retrieve and summarize published articles, and help create documents. Salaries for the junior staff are generally in the range from $40,000 to $50,000, although with time and experience they can advance up the ranks depending mainly on their ability to work independently and do high quality work. In the middle of the organizational structure is the majority of the professional staff who provide the specific expertise needed to attract clients and accomplish what is often highly technical work.

Our company, for example, has various staff experts in the production of clinical trial reports, statistical data analysis, control of drug manufacturing, evaluation of animal toxicology results, and so forth. Most of the staff brings some extent of postgraduate training or relevant industry experience and often some prior experience with consulting. Those less experienced, who can be used broadly because they are bright and capable but may not be sufficiently knowledgeable in any given area to be handed much autonomy with clients, are generally paid in the range from $80,000 to $90,000. Those more experienced, especially with specialized postgraduate training and/or extensive industry background, serve as the company "experts" in their given field. Because of their preconsulting professional background and knowledge, these are high-level consultants who author many of the reports and serve as client contacts much of the time. Such staff members generally are paid between $125,000 and $150,000, depending greatly on whether they provide very specific expertise and depending on their track record for bringing in business. For these mid-level staff, advancement into the practice director tier of our company is dependent exclusively on marketing prowess: how many new clients has one been bringing in and how much revenue is involved.

The Daily Routine, or More Accurately, Nonroutine

A typical day begins with an attempt to triage work on several projects. There are usually strict deadlines for some projects and flexible deadlines for others, so it is generally possible to prioritize. I most often have two or three projects going simultaneously, but sometimes I have more. On a good day, all is quiet and it's possible to concentrate solely on the work at hand. On a bad day, there may be a rapidly approaching deadline, a series of phone calls, and scheduled and unscheduled client meetings. Generally,

Murphy's Law conspires to make the busy bad days as complex as possible, and the morning triage of work undergoes adjustment as necessary.

Many of my projects involve a team of 3 to 10 people, each team member contributing a defined role toward the project outcome based on area of expertise. These group projects occupy most of my time—I would estimate that less than 20% of my time is spent on individual projects. Luckily, e-mail makes collaborative projects a snap. In my particular case, with the main office of my company three time zones away to the east, the interactive work takes place during the earlier portions of the day, whereas much of the individual project work gets accomplished after the rest of the firm has gone home for the evening. Of course, the bicoastal nature of my company's offices and the majority of our clients being located on the east coast ensure that 5:00 A.M. teleconferences are part of the price we of the San Francisco contingent pay to live where we do.

A scientific consulting company the size and scope of ours makes money by developing a top reputation and doing excellent work, having many clients and paying jobs at all times, billing as many hours as possible by as many employees as possible, and placing a major focus on marketing. Therefore, the days tend to be full, with essentially nonstop work most of the time. The hours tend to be reasonable (probably an average of 40 to 50 hours per week), with a good deal of flexibility, potential for working from home, and so forth. Many of us eat our lunches at our desks while we are working on projects (we look at this as a health benefit rather than loss of a lunch hour).

With electronic sharing by e-mail and the growing popularity of video-conferencing, the vast quantity of our work, even the complicated collaborative projects, is usually done from our own desks. Some of our larger projects have impossibly tight deadlines confined by external factors, such as scheduled meetings at FDA. For the most part, however, we have enough time to do a job right without working all night or weekend. In a company the size of ours, there can easily be 50 to 100 or more active projects, so the operational term for most of us is multitasking. While this can cause some uncomfortable juggling at crunch times, it is a very efficient way to stay motivated and intellectually engaged.

What Makes the Job Fun and What Makes It Tough

In our firm, people are turned on for various reasons. The CEO is excited by the firm's reputation as a solver of the most difficult problems. Others are excited by their success in marketing the firm and bringing in business. For me, it is the variety of projects and predominance of truly challenging tasks that constitute the greatest source of enjoyment and helps keep the job fresh. The rewards are many: I put all my training and scientific/medical knowledge to much greater use than I ever did in academia, I get paid to think a lot, and I am forced to learn something new for many of my projects. There is a tremendous amount of professional growth in a job like mine, and with the ever-changing face of science and medicine, it is hard to envision projects ever getting old and stale.

I find the greatest challenge to be the marketing aspects of the consulting business. Considerable effort needs to be expended on getting introductions to new prospective clients, finding out if they have problems we could help with, and of course convincing them it is in their best interest to hire us. In some respects, the work harkens back to the situation in academic research whereby you may write 10 grants to get one funded: a lot of effort goes unrewarded. For the natural marketers of the firm, this process and its rewards are a tremendous source of satisfaction. For others of us, myself included, it is a necessary evil—part of the process of getting a fun and challenging project to tackle.

A FOCUS ON BUSINESS DEVELOPMENT

A consulting firm like ours depends on finding new clients and having old clients come back to us time and again. Although some acquisition of new clients is accomplished by advertising, most client attraction comes from one-on-one marketing. Some of the larger consulting companies may have a dedicated business development function, and the technical staff is tasked with simply getting the work done. However, most firms like ours use the high-level expertise of our professional staff to further market the firm, as well as to work on projects. The rub is that only the time spent working on projects (i.e., billable work) directly brings revenue to the firm. Consequently, we are constantly striving to balance efforts to maximize billability and at the same time develop new business. Most of the time, these efforts can be juggled successfully. However, during the times when we are overwhelmed with projects, it is difficult to make the time and have the discipline to maintain marketing efforts. On the flip side, when business is slow and marketing efforts are critical, it is hard not to feel overly anxious and pressured.

For many who are new to the consulting world, the necessity for acting like a salesperson is one of the greatest adjustments when coming from the ivory tower. Many of us science-types have little or no prior experience in marketing and tend to think we have little aptitude. With time, though, we all gain marketing experience, and most of us find we have more aptitude than we thought. The other significant adjustment is keeping an even keel during the down times when business is slow. In the lab, you can always keep yourself busy by doing more experiments, but it is much more difficult to feel productive as a consultant when you cannot keep busy with paying business.

WOULD YOU MAKE A GOOD BIOMEDICAL CONSULTANT?

I believe the most important qualities for a scientific consultant to succeed in a firm like ours are the ability to listen and to think creatively. This is because very little of what we do is "cookie-cutter" work. We don't have canned reports or canned analyses just waiting for data to be plugged in, and we don't have a standard approach for problems. A perfect example is the product due diligence project, in which some clients require only a relatively brief review for potential problems ("red flags"), whereas others demand a very detailed, thoughtful analysis taking into account all the pros and cons so that as informed a judgment as possible can be made. These are very different approaches, with very different degrees of effort and expense.

> "I believe the most important qualities for a scientific consultant to succeed in a firm like ours are the ability to listen and to think creatively."

It is critical that you listen to the client and understand what is needed. There are several possible pitfalls if you misunderstand the client's needs and misinterpret the assignment. In one instance, you may try to sell an in-depth due diligence report that covers all the bases, but what the client requires is a high-level overview because the detailed diligence has already been completed. In this instance, the potential client will likely laugh at your proposal and go elsewhere. In another instance, a project may require the analysis of a rocket scientist (assume the firm doesn't have one), but you fail to understand that this level of expertise is required. Consequently, your report may prove superficial and totally inadequate, and the client won't come back. Alternatively, if clients underestimate their risk, for instance believing that their potential FDA issue is relatively negligible when a very real alternative outcome is to be put out of business, it is critical that you listen carefully and ask enough questions to make the distinction. Each of these scenarios illustrates the importance of defining the client's issue and proposing an appropriate approach to solving the problem.

The other feature of a good consultant is being able to think creatively. Although occasionally there are right answers and wrong answers regarding a client's problem, this is usually not the case in my world. For most of my projects, there is the need to integrate information, form judgments, and/or create scientifically supportable arguments; one can't simply go to a book and find the "correct" answer. Creative approaches also are necessary when the client's need is to persuade someone, such as an FDA regulator or a trial judge, of the merit of the client's perspective. These types of projects often involve a mix of building support for the client's point of view while simultaneously producing evidence to counteract the perspective that puts the client at risk. One of the most satisfying statements a consultant can hear from a client is "You know, I never thought of that."

ADVICE ON BECOMING A BIOMEDICAL CONSULTANT

I came directly from academia to consulting. It was a relatively smooth transition, in large part due to my considerable postgraduate training and academic experience that immediately could be put to work on projects. With the broad range of scientific and biomedical assignments we undertake at our firm, I didn't need a great deal of on-the-job training. For those of you with a similarly extensive academic background, you'd probably be surprised how much you could contribute immediately in the consulting world.

For those of you more recently out of college or graduate training, a direct jump into consulting similarly is an option, although it doesn't afford you the greatest leverage. An alternative approach would be to get experience first in a relevant industry setting. For example, if you are interested in pharmaceutical consulting, a stint in a drug company, in a contract research organization (CRO), or at the FDA would be invaluable experience, and the background you would gain could be immediately applicable for consulting. Similarly, time spent with the Environmental Protection Agency or a state agency would give you instant credibility and relevant experience for environmental/toxicology consulting. Relevant industry experience not only is extremely useful for obtaining technical expertise, but it also can increase your value in the marketing arena. Many of our clients chose our company because so-and-so worked in regulatory at a pharmaceutical company or because so-and-so was at the FDA.

Learning more about biomedical consulting is best achieved by talking directly with people in the industry. There aren't any relevant industry organizations, newsletters, or meetings on the national scale to give you a flavor of the occupation. However, depending on your locale, there may well be regional consultant groups that have periodic networking meetings. Consulting groups, large and small, can usually be identified by searching the Web, and a few phone calls will generally provide you with information about regional networking groups. Once you have a networking roster and begin to attend meetings, you can readily get answers to your questions and feedback on your credentials.

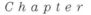

Chapter

15

∙∙∙∙∙∙∙∙∙∙

SALES AND MARKETING:

So You Want to Sell?

∙∙∙∙∙∙∙∙∙∙∙∙∙∙∙∙∙

Erin Hall Meade, R.M., S.M., F.A.A.M.

Head of Development and Public Education, Life Alaska Donor Services

Former Pacific Northwest Sales Manager, LAS Laboratories (ret.)

My name is Erin Hail Meade, and I was the Pacific Northwest Sales Manager for LAS Laboratories, one of the largest environmental testing labs in the nation. I am now working with Life Alaska Donor Services in public relations and development. I have an honors B.S. degree in medical microbiology, with a minor in chemistry. I made it through all the course work and lab work for a Ph.D. in medical microbiology and infectious diseases, and I am a Registered Specialist Microbiologist. Although I sat on the board of the National Registry of Microbiologists for several years and am a Fellow of the American Academy of Microbiologists, I have never worked as a laboratory microbiologist. I have been in technical sales for the past 18 years, and I *love* it.

HOW DID I GET HERE?

In 1980, I had just passed my qualifying oral exams for my doctorate in micro-biology. Ahead of me loomed 6 months of working in a small, windowless room, refining my piles of research into an acceptable dissertation. Somehow, I was uninspired by the prospect.

That night, I lost even more of my motivation when I opened the *Journal of Bacteriology* and looked at the post-doctoral positions listed in the back. The salaries were between $8000 and $11,000 per year, barely living wages, even for an ex-grad student used to living on the financial edge. About 2 days later, while I was still stewing over my impending fate, a friend called and told me that a small chemistry laboratory in the San Francisco Bay area was looking for a lab manager and paying $18,000 a year. I walked away from the dissertation and never regretted it.

I spent a year with that first company. When it went bankrupt, I jumped to its largest competitor, again as lab manager, for a 50% increase in salary. I lasted there for 5 years, then was "laid off." (Actually, I was fired because I was in the wrong political camp during a power shift. Oh, well.) I noticed that the *only* people not canned were the salespeople! When I asked why, I was told, "They're too valuable to lose—they are the ones bringing in all the money!" The point was well taken.

I quickly began looking for a sales job, but I kept hearing the same comments. "You're too smart, so you'll talk over people's heads." "You have no sales experience." "Technical types can't do sales, they're too arrogant, and they lack the common touch." "How do you know you can do sales, anyway?" All were valid points.

I started looking for a company that would train me to do sales, one that specifically advertised "no experience needed." I expected to take a drop in salary at first—and I certainly did. In 1984, I went from $50,000 per year to $35,000 per year and gave up a company car. However, I did learn to do outside sales and found that I loved it.

I loved the freedom of making my own hours; I loved the challenge of selling something technical to other techno-weenies like myself, and

• • • • • • • • • • • • • • • • • • • •
"I loved the challenge of selling something technical to other techno-weenies like myself, and I loved winning."
• • • • • • • • • • • • • • • • • • • •

I loved winning. Losing was no great shakes, but I soon learned not to dwell on the losses—they would be wins next time, I decided. I also loved the money; salespeople are often some of the highest paid people in a company, and rightly so—they are the main funnels for cash into the business. Of course, the other employees are equally valuable. But, frankly, they are not perceived as such by the people making most of the salary decisions. The job security is excellent—why would you lay off someone bringing in roughly 10 to 20 times their gross salary every year? (And, by the way, this is a good rule of thumb for a salesperson to calculate what they should be earning—figure you need to sell 10 to 20 times what you make in gross salary, including all benefits and perquisites.)

●●●●●●●●●●●●●●●●●●●●●●●●
"I didn't sell anything high tech in that first sales job; in fact, I sold some pretty disgusting stuff"
●●●●●●●●●●●●●●●●●●●●●●●●

I didn't sell anything high tech in that first sales job; in fact, I sold some pretty disgusting stuff (industrial maintenance chemicals used for exciting applications such as cleaning grease traps for french fry machines at McDonalds). But I got good at it by paying attention, working 14 hours a day, reading all the company literature that no one else read, and doing a lot of planning and strategizing before I left the house every morning.

So, I learned to do sales, lasted 1½ years, and jumped into a technical sales job in another company working in a technical field—environmental laboratory services. I wanted to sell something interesting and sell to more intellectually challenging clients than those buying cleaning solutions. I immediately jumped back to $50,000, got a company car again, and was selling something high tech that was way cool. I was feeling good. Face it—you didn't sit in school for 16 to 24 years to be satisfied selling nontech stuff that is part of a commodity market. This type of sales does not challenge you and does not really let you use all those cool resources you've accrued over the years. Selling technically interesting things (or services) forces you to use your brain, draw on all the knowledge you've accumulated, and *be there* all the time.

A technical degree (or two or three) gives you two distinct advantages over the other salespeople in your field. First, it teaches you to think on your feet, to look at loads of information and identify the salient components needed to answer the clients' questions, and to distinguish between useful and garbage information. Second, most of your competition is hiring sales reps with nontechnical backgrounds, who sell by the "Hey, buddy, how about them Niners?" technique. While this approach can work in certain settings, most clients buying pharmaceuticals, laboratory services, or some other specialized service will be greatly annoyed by it. Few, if any, of my clients want to talk about the big game.

When a client asked me a technical question, I didn't have to say, "I don't know; I'll have to ask someone *smart* and get back to you." Instead, I said, "Sure, you can pick up phenols in a standard GCMS scan; which ones do you need to see?" This ability to grasp the question and come up with a useful answer saved my client time and often led to my selling even more services than the client originally anticipated buying.

Not only do I use my scientific background even today, but I also use the abilities covertly installed in me during school not to get distracted by extraneous information, to meet deadlines and budgets *no matter what*, and to make the extra effort to ensure everything is done perfectly.

WHAT DO I DO?

For my previous job at LAS, I sold environmental testing services for one of the largest environmental testing laboratories in the nation. My territory included all areas from Fresno, California, to the North Pole, and from the Pacific Ocean east to Boise, Idaho. This sounds like a large territory—and it is—but there are only about seven key cities in it, which is where I focused most of my attention.

I traveled a *lot*—about 3 weeks out of 4, on average. I learned to live out of a suitcase and learned to enjoy it. In fact, after all this time, I can't imagine opening my eyes every morning to the same scenery. How dull.

• •

"I traveled a lot—about 3 weeks out of 4, on average. I learned to live out of a suitcase and learned to enjoy it."

• •

I made client calls on both new and existing clients; I wrote quotes, bids, and proposals; I reviewed contracts prior to sending them to the legal department (so I could spot problems early in the game and often defuse them before they become deal-stoppers); I helped clients sort out problems; and I kept *extensive* records, so if I was hit by a bus, someone could step in and take over my territory with minimal hassle.

Part of the reason for good record keeping is that the environmental testing industry is driven by state and federal regulations. Few companies would choose voluntarily to spend $50,000 to $500,000 per year just to monitor their environmental messes. Therefore, the federal government has made it a legal requirement to do so.

The salesperson is often in the middle of a huge web of regulations, requirements, suggestions, and just plain field realities that need to be sorted out, coordinated, and pulled back together to make the project work. Which regulations apply first? How do you meet the needs of multiple regulators, field personnel, accountants, engineers, and lab people while still making sure everyone plays nice with each other? The case can be made that this is not the salesperson's problem. Fine, I agree . . . . Of course, then nothing gets done, or it gets done wrong, or the client is unhappy, and the regulator is unhappy; at this point, you're in trouble. So, it is necessary to rethink this idea. Whose responsibility is it to make sure everything goes well? *Yours.*

You're handling problems from both sides; your company (those wonderful folks that say to you, "You sell it; we'll take care of making it, doing it, designing it, and implementing it.") has been known to let you down. ("Gee, it was my day off . . . I don't know where the fax went, but I never got it. . .Well, we've been *very* busy lately, and it must just have slipped through the cracks.") Then you are in the unenviable position of selling the problem to the client: "No, it's not really a problem; it's an *opportunity for personal growth.*"

How Much Do I Make?

There are five ways in which salespeople can be paid; you can usually get a combination of these.

Salary

Salary can be regarded as a flat rate, paid in weekly, fortnightly, or monthly increments; it increases only when you get a raise, usually only once or twice a year. The advantage is that a salary is dependable. You always know from month to month what your financial baseline will be. Salary varies with the job, the company, and its expectations of you. An entry-level technical salesperson typically will get from $45,000 to $50,000 to start. Someone with around 5 years of relevant experience and a good track record should look for at least $50,000 to $75,000. A senior sales rep with a good track record of sales should expect from $65,000 to $120,000 annually. If you're in a hot industry, you can make a lot more.

Commission

Commission is a percentage of the revenue income that you bring into the company through your sales activities. Avoid a "commission-only" position, particularly if you're just starting in a job. Usually it takes several months to establish a client base in a new position and get sales revenues up to a meaningful level. If you receive only commission, you'll be working for very little income (sometimes no income, if the company has a revenue cap that must be exceeded for commission to kick in) until that point.

As you become established, commission is a good way to go—it gives you a way to determine your own income based on your selling skills, the amount of time you put into the job, and the real value of the products you're selling.

Commission-only settings are best left to the seasoned sales reps, who have a realistic idea of their sales abilities, an established client base, and can continue to sell successfully month after month. But even as a beginning sales rep, you are bringing value to the company other than revenue. You're advertising for the company that hired you, and you're building client contacts and name recognition for the company that will last long after you are gone. Because the company gains intangibles from your activities, it should pay you some baseline salary that underlies your commission, to keep you going until the commissions start.

Base Salary

A base salary is the minimal amount people on a commission plan get from the company, on a regular basis, to handle basic support. This is usually anywhere from $45,000 to $65,000 annually. Commissions are added on to this amount.

Draw

A draw is an amount of money a company gives you to get you started. Be very careful—*it is only a loan* and will be repaid out of your commissions (when they start), or, if you quit, it is often repaid out of your pocket. When a company uses a draw to get you going, you're essentially working for free, as in the commission-only scenario. This is rarely a good idea.

Bonus

A bonus is the happy event that occurs on an irregular or regular basis and is a monetary reward for doing something particularly well—exceeding your sales quota, landing a particularly good account, or helping the entire team have a good sales period. Bonuses are a great incentive—they're a slug of cash all at once and really perk up your day! Always ask, when you're hired, if your plan includes a bonus and how you can qualify for it. Get the bonus plan in writing so everyone is on the same page when it comes time to cut a check.

Perquisites

Perquisites are the nifty little "gimmes" that are partially or totally nontaxable or nonreportable (by you) and that make life nicer. Examples include a company car, a gasoline credit card or cell phone for which the company pays, a laptop or desktop computer that the company buys, an expense account, and so forth (like the right to keep all your frequent flyer miles, which can translate into neat, cheap vacations).

> *"Perquisites are the nifty little "gimmes" that are particularly or totally nontaxable or nonreportable (by you) and that make life nicer."*

The best part is that Uncle Sam gets little or none of this stuff because it is not really cash, and it is not really given to you—you are just using it to do work for the company. It is important to remember that perquisites should never be abused, or they can disappear (often, along with your job). Don't use your car phone to order take-out pizza or use your company credit card to take your mom to dinner. However, you *can* use your credit card to take a client to dinner—as long as you discuss business during that time.

Similarly, you cannot drive the company car across the country for a family reunion without reporting this as "income" on your taxes (and, to the company, as "personal use," if that is allowed), but you can use it to drive to another city to visit a client and (happy coincidence!) your best friend, who happens to live in the same city. If you are smart, remain honest, and play by the rules, all of this will work out wonderfully.

Extra Options

Some firms, particularly start-ups, can't afford a senior sales rep but truly need one. In this case, they may offer stock or partial ownership in lieu of a juicy salary. This is a judgment call—you're gambling that the company will become hugely successful and that you'll make your money back in spades. Go with your gut feeling. If you think this technology is the greatest thing since crunchy peanut butter, then do it. However, if it's a "me, too" technology, is half-baked, or otherwise smells a little whiffy, politely decline. Cash in your pocket is often better than founder's stock that matures in 7 years (and in which you vest in 5 years); you're betting today's earnings against stock performance 5 to 10 years in the future.

HOW DO YOU PREPARE FOR THIS SORT OF CAREER?

The big catch-22 is that you can't get a sales job until you have sales experience, but you can't get sales experience until they hire you to do sales—right? Wrong. You can take a job as an in-house sales representative (entry-level position, usually involving phone work), do that for a year or so, and learn sales that way—plus you can show the company what you can do. You can also get a job in client support/customer service, supporting the sales department, and learn that way. Or, look for a company that is willing to train you, as long as you swear to work for them for a certain amount of time once training is complete. Any of these approaches work well. My estimate is that you'll spend from 1 to 2 years in inside sales, 1 to 2 years in low-level outside sales, and then you're totally out on your own—a terrific place to be.

Is it necessary to know something about an industry to sell for it? Yes . . . and no. Knowing something about the industry can help you get a foot in the door, can give you an advantage over other job applicants, can help you manage your sales territory for the first few months, and can help you target the appropriate accounts right off the bat. However, you'll really do 99% of your learning on the job. I had *zero* knowledge about each industry when I first started. I paid attention, sold my sales and/or management skills over my knowledge of the industry, and learned fast. It worked for me.

The typical promotion pathway often looks like this:

Inside sales (i.e., phone sales) → outside sales, junior grade → outside sales → product manager → sales manager → director of sales → vice president of sales

Note that inside phone sales *is not* telemarketing. You do not annoy people by calling them at dinnertime; you sit in the company office and answer phone calls from new or existing clients who need information or wish to place an order. Inside sales is the bottom of the ladder—you have a tough job, you have to show up in the office, and you have to dress appropriately. You need to be on time on a daily basis, and people yell at you over the phone; you never get to meet anyone face-to-face, which makes it much harder to develop a relationship with your client, and the money is not great. The good news is that it doesn't last forever. Think of it as your internship.

Outside sales, junior grade, means that you often travel with a senior person who shows you the ropes. This allows you to learn a lot in a short time. While the money isn't great, it's better than inside sales.

Becoming a product manager may or may not be a promotion. When you're a product manager, you have the responsibility of building name recognition and a client base for one particular product, but you don't sell anything else, which can be limiting and can cut you off from your former client base. However, if you make a new product a huge success, you get all sorts of money and recognition within the company, which is good for promotability.

Becoming sales director is the holy grail for some salespeople, while others prefer to lay low and live the good life as a field salesperson. Personality usually determines whether you will want to go to this stage. Being a director means you spend your time managing salespeople, who are also known as "cowboys" because of their cussedness and independence. After being a manager for 5 years, I gratefully dropped back into being a salesperson—so the only person I had to manage was myself. And, contrary to common belief, being the manager does not necessarily mean more money—just more aggravation.

Becoming vice president of sales means you take the headaches of being sales director, multiply them tenfold, and then add corporate politics on top. Personally, I have no interest in this position. However, the money is really good—expect to make $150,000 to $250,000 annually, with performance bonuses on top of that. If you're in a hot company, you can do even better.

CAREER MOBILITY

If you get tired of sales and decide to switch careers or companies, you should know that a good sales rep can go just about anywhere, given the proper network. Selling is an innate talent as well as a trainable skill, and not everyone can do it. This makes you valuable. You can switch companies easily, switch industries with a bit more effort, and with diligence move to a very senior position in a corporation. A majority of CEOs in Fortune 500 companies formerly were sales reps, according to *Forbes Magazine.*

The key here is *who you know*—networking is everything. The higher up a sales position is, the less likely it is to be advertised, and the more likely it is to be filled by connections, networking, and word of mouth. Never overlook headhunters (kindly known as "recruiters" or "search consultants")—some of the best jobs are found through them because they can winnow through the chaff looking for the truly golden individual for a particular opportunity. *Always* be nice to headhunters—they are good nodes in your network. When they call you, be polite and listen, even if you don't think you are interested. If it's not the right job for you, say so—and then suggest someone else you know who might be a better fit. The headhunters don't forget favors like this. They also call you more often, and thus you are more likely to hear about a truly nifty job.

WHAT ABOUT TRAVEL?

Sales absolutely requires an enormous amount of travel. There is a direct correlation between the sales revenues I bring in and the amount of time I am sitting in front of a client. Phone calls, e-mails, and even video conferencing do not bring in the same results. Just the idea that you thought enough of someone to get on an airplane to come see them warms the cockles of even the hardest heart—especially if you do it regularly.

I traveled about 3 weeks every month, hitting all seven of the major cities in my sales territory (in California—San Jose, San Francisco, East Bay, and Sacramento; in Washington—Seattle and Richland; and in Alaska—Anchorage). I logged about 100,000 airplane miles per year. You really do get used to it. In fact, there are some tricks for making it down-right enjoyable.

For example, I'd find one hotel in every town, and I always stayed there. I got to know the staff, the best rooms, the concierges, and (especially) the reservations manager. Whenever I went to that city, I called the reservations manager and told him or her that I was coming back to the hotel for a few days. I got the best rooms for the lowest rates, and people were always happy to see me. In return, I gave them all my business in that city; I *always* wrote a thank-you card to the reservations manager after I left, and I tried to remember key people's names. People *love* to hear their name—it is the loveliest sound in the world to them. (See, I am always selling!)

Another tip—buy a good map of a city (*not* a rental car map!) and keep it in a file where you keep all the other pertinent information on that city, including client locations, dry cleaners, hotels, drug stores, and so on. Then, when you get ready to visit that city, just grab the file and throw it in your briefcase. You will become so familiar with the city that, after a few trips, it feels just like home. I learned to like Anchorage so much that I moved there.

Try to fly with only one airline, whenever you can. You not only rack up miles (leading to preferential treatment and first-class upgrades), you also get to know the gate people—which can come in very handy when a flight is oversold, if you have excess luggage, if you're running late, or for any number of other little problems that life or the TSA may throw your way.

Learn to pack a suitcase properly. Everyone knows how to pack, right? Wrong. For 5 days out, a woman will need two jackets, five blouses/shirts, and one dark skirt or pants. Period. You need one pair of jeans for night, to wear with the same blouse you wore during the day. Bring one pair of shoes—low heels or flats—that match the skirt or pants. You also need one purse to match the shoes and one nightgown. I bring one pair of running shoes, just for walking around after work.

I leave the rest up to you, but remember—you're probably not going to run into Prince Charles, so don't bring anything extra because it just adds weight. I can go out for 5 days with one small carry-on suitcase. I toured mainland China for 4 weeks with carry-on luggage and did just fine. There are department stores everywhere, and it takes 5 minutes to pick up an extra pair of panty hose or clean socks. And 24-hour dry cleaners exist, so a coffee stain on a jacket is no big deal—just switch to the second jacket for a day.

WHAT COMPANIES HAVE SALESPEOPLE?

Easy—*all* companies have salespeople. Some companies have different names for them—account representatives, business development personnel, marketing representatives, and so on. Any company that sells a thing, an idea, or a service has to have someone to sell it for them. And it might as well be you!

What percentage of a company is composed of salespeople? This can vary widely, depending on what they sell. My lab had 75 to 90 employees. We had four salespeople, and we brought in $9 million to $14 million a year—enough to keep those 90 people employed. If a company is just a "shell" (meaning it is just a middleman, adding cost but relatively little other value to someone else's product other than a sales force), the percentage of employees who are in sales can be as high as 90%. However, watch out for this type of company—it usually doesn't take good care of its salespeople, and its clients can often cut the sales team out and go directly to the source of the goods or service, thus cutting out the mark-up.

Also, watch out for companies that sell commodity items; if it sells boring stuff, then *anyone* who can walk and breathe simultaneously can sell it. This "stuff" refers to office supplies, copiers, telephone systems, encyclopedias, maintenance chemicals, paper supplies, restaurant supplies, and other such items. If it doesn't take any special skills, intelligence, or talent to sell the product, you are in stiff competition with the 23-year-old buxom blonde who giggles and snaps her gum but is cute as hell—and she's going to get that sale almost every time. It sounds trite, but it's true. Try to sell something that takes brains to understand and explain—there's less competition, you have better job security, and it's a lot more challenging intellectually. Plus, you become more valuable to the company as you get older, not less valuable.

WHAT SKILLS ARE NECESSARY?

It is critical that you have the ability to meet people and become comfortable with them easily. You also need the ability to talk to strangers and an ability to accept criticism and rejection without taking it personally. Just because they don't buy your product doesn't mean you're a bad person; they're just not buying the product from you. No big deal, just go find someone else who *will* buy from you.

You will need to be completely self-motivated, especially in outside sales. No one from your company sees you regularly, no one tells you to get out of bed and make an 8:00 A.M. appointment, and no one watches to see what time you quit in the evening—it is all entirely up to you. This can be a fatal trap for someone who is not internally motivated because, while no one is watching you, they are all watching your numbers. If your sales fall below average, you're soon on the street again—with no reference for your next job.

You will also need to be exceptionally well organized because you will keep your own files. When I was a salesperson for LAS, I spent 1 day per week just on paperwork—writing quotes and proposals, filing quotes, responding to requests for information; tracking procurements and projects; keeping up with time cards, expense reports, and mileage logs, and dealing with tracking customer problems. When I was out of town for 2 to 3 weeks, I would spend the first 3 days back at home just playing paperwork catch-up.

You also need to have good time management skills. You have to get everything done in a reasonable amount of time or else your job will engulf you and eat up your entire life. Sales takes a lot of time—I worked an average of 10 hours a day—but it also gives you the ability to manage your time however you want. I might have played hooky one afternoon to climb a glacier while in Alaska, but I'd work until 11:30 P.M. the next night writing a proposal that was due the following day. There were days I worked 4 hours, then quit to lie in the sun; but there were many more days when I worked until after dinnertime.

You must be able to write easily and well because you will be doing a great deal of it—proposals, bids, reports, letters, and so on. If writing is a struggle for you, sales is not your field—you must leave a clear paper trail behind you, for both legal and professional reasons.

Being a confident, aggressive person is a plus. A shrinking violet has a hard time in sales. While confidence comes with time and knowledge of your product and your company, the inherent ability to walk up to a stranger and say, "Hi, I'm Erin Hall Meade, and I work for LAS Laboratories. Can I talk to you for 5 minutes?" is mandatory. Never be embarrassed—if things don't work out, you just walk away and they'll forget you in no time.

Many people say good looks are important in outside sales. Although it is true that everyone likes to look at handsome people, this is *not* a job requirement. It is more important that you have a pleasant personality, that you are well groomed, and that you are confident (does this sound like something you heard in your high school health class?). A well-dressed, personable individual will always come out ahead of a gorgeous airhead hunk (unless you are selling copiers or carpet shampoo, and why would you want to do that?). Many people in the sales field (with other companies) have minimal technical training. I had no difficulty selling against them, even though they may have been younger, better looking, thinner, and so on. When a client would say, "How can I do this job for the least money, getting the best data?" the airhead would say, "I'll call my office and get a technical person to call you back." I said, "Let me show you how to optimize this project, saving both time and money." My success rate was higher than average because I knew my field and the technology, not because I was the best-looking person in the field (which, of course, I was. Ha!).

WHAT DOES A TYPICAL DAY LOOK LIKE?

I had two types of days: on the road and in the office.

In the Office

Most of the time, my office was in my home, which worked out very well for me. At about 7:15 or 7:30 A.M., I checked my phone messages on one line, while checking my e-mail on another. While I was doing this, I also pulled my faxes from the night before off the facsimile machine. I took 15 to 30 minutes to note the things I needed to do that day, with A, B, or C priorities. I also checked to see what I did not finish the day before and added it to this list, again with appropriate priorities included.

At about 8:00 A.M., I rolled my telephone off the night line so that it rang instead of going to voice mail. I didn't do this earlier because otherwise I'd never get any planning done first. I continued to answer all voice messages, e-mail, and faxes. Then, I began calling clients to make future appointments, resolve problems, follow up on proposals and quotes, catch up on local industry gossip, and reinforce relationships with key clients.

After this was done, I wrote reports, filled out time cards, car logs, expense reports, and other paperwork. During the entire day, I handled phone calls from clients, lab people, other sales reps, government regulators, and so on. I usually did my filing just before I quit for the night, which was between 4:30 and 7:30 P.M.

On the Road

I never went on a road trip without having at least 50% of my sales calls already scheduled with clients. I used a cell phone to make the rest of them while I was driving between sales calls. I wrote reports, answered e-mail, and got faxes in my hotel at night. I checked my voice mail by cell phone 10 to 15 times each day; I don't like to let more than an hour elapse between receiving a message and returning the call. I often ate dinner in my room, so I could catch up on paperwork, faxes, and so on. I got a lot of reading done as well.

WHAT ARE THE PROS AND CONS OF THE JOB?

I *love* the freedom, the fun, and the adrenaline rushes when I win the sale. I love the travel (especially on someone else's nickel), love the challenge, love meeting new people, enjoy seeing new places, and like learning new things daily. I am a true adrenaline junkie—I love the ups and downs of sales. And, best of all, my job is just plain *fun* much of the time. Gee, and they pay me a lot of money for this! Wow!

I *don't* like it when I'm not in control over things that affect my clients, especially problems in my company's lab that impact its ability to get the work done well and on time. I can't sell in the field and direct things in the laboratory at the same time. Sometimes I feel like a mushroom—the lab keeps me in the dark and feeds me manure. I find out about a problem with a client often after the client does—I hate this. Still, it happens. I have to deal with it and do damage control wherever possible. This means that I have to maintain a decent relationship with the people at my company to keep them responsive to my concerns about my clients. I often have to convince them to do my clients' work before they do someone else's work. In that way, the people inside my company are also my "clients." I have to sell them on the idea of doing my outside clients' work first.

It was easy for me to get used to managing my own time; after all, that's what you do in grad school. No one checks to see if you're going to class, but you'd better do well on the exams or you're sunk. I also had no difficulty getting used to making on-the-spot decisions, sometimes involving hundreds of thousands of dollars. Once I feel I have the technical knowledge to make the right decision, I just do what seems best—and, most of the time, I'm right. When I'm wrong, I face it, and it's okay. I've never been fired for making a bad decision, but you can certainly get fired for not making a decision at all.

How Often Do I Have a Hair-on-Fire Day?

Fairly often, maybe 25% of the time, I have a crazy day. As I mentioned earlier, I am an adrenaline junkie, so I go for the highs and lows. I *love* days when I have 20 hours of things to do and only 15 hours in which to do them—this is when I'm at my most creative, productive, and stressed out. These 15 hours fly by in minutes—I don't eat, I lose track of time, and I love it. If you are not into pressure and stress, you may not like sales. But I always feel something is happening!

> "If you are not into pressure and stress, you may not like sales. But I always feel something is happening!"

I am a perfectionist. I love to win. I want my clients to know they can always count on me to be their advocate in the lab. I want them to see me as a technical resource, and I want them to know that I will always advise them about the best way to spend their money, even if it's not with my company on a particular job. In fact, one of the best ways to build credibility with a long-term client is to tell them how to spend less or how to spend it with one of your competitors. As long as this is truly the best thing for them at the time, they'll remember you as the one who told them the truth, and they'll always come back.

Finally, think technically! You have had tons of education, you have had tons of training to help you gather and sort through data and synthesize solutions from mountains of information, and you have been trained to *think on your feet*. These are skills many other people don't have, so let these work for you. And have fun.

WHAT I HAVE BEEN DOING FOR 7 YEARS

I retired from the field of technical sales in 1999 and fulfilled a lifelong dream by moving to Anchorage, Alaska. I now head the development (developing a network of financial donors) and public education (public relations) programs for Life Alaska Donor Services, the nonprofit organ and tissue bank for the state of Alaska. I see this position as simply another sales and marketing job, albeit for a higher purpose.

FROM DOING RESEARCH TO MOVING RESEARCH:

My Life in Tech Transfer

· · · · · · · · · · · · · · · ·

Paula Szoka, Ph.D.

Director, Invention Licensing, University of Washington Technology Transfer

While my career path has tracked through a wide range of job titles, it has not been nearly as random as it may look at first glance. I have always planned out what I wanted to do in my life. With each new task, my goal was to try it for about 5 years and see if I could achieve certain benchmarks. If yes, then I'd stay. If not . . . it was time for the next step down the path. As it turned out, my family and my own ambitions together dictated the career decisions that I made throughout my career.

· ·

"With each new task, my goal was to try it for about 5 years and see if I could achieve certain benchmarks. If yes, then I'd stay. If not . . . it was time for the next step down the path."

· ·

I decided at an early age to be a scientist—back in eighth grade, in fact. My entire education was geared toward becoming a research scientist with a Ph.D. After finishing graduate school and facing the almost total lack of tenure track positions, my ambitions were relatively small. I didn't want to end up running a big lab, but I did want to be my own boss. Thus, I headed down the classic post-doctoral path.

My daughter was born right as I finished graduate school (I got pregnant on schedule, but she showed up ahead of time!), and my husband was in a tenure-track position at NY State University in Buffalo. So my first postdoc position was in the lab where I did my graduate work.

When that first post-doc was completed, I moved to MIT with my daughter in tow. My husband had a faculty position at NY State for the first year while we were in Boston, then landed a faculty position at Tufts, so we were at least in the same state! My lab director did not like having a "single" mom in the lab, so I moved to Massachusetts General Hospital/Harvard for a 2-year stint.

Just as we started to settle in, my husband's department chairman left Tufts. He felt that the new chair would probably want to refocus the research within the department, and so he took a position at the University of California, San Francisco, in late 1980. I decided that three post-doc positions were enough, and I set out to find a job instead.

OFF TO THE CORPORATE WORLD

At that time, academic scientists disdained industry as having second-rate research and looked down on those of us who left the ivory tower for the corporate world. I started at Syntex Corporation (Palo Alto, California) on Halloween 1980, with the idea of giving it my best shot for 5 years and seeing if I could reach my goals in molecular biology research. By the time I was 3 years into it, it was very obvious this would not make me happy. I had a horrible boss who basically used me as a glorified technician; the company gave lip service to but not real support for a company policy that allowed researchers to spend 20% of their time on original work. I spent the last 2 years of that job actively looking to change my career path.

As luck would have it, Syntex had excellent programs to help employees do just that without needing to leave the company, including personality profiling, management training in running meetings, time and stress management, training sessions on principals of supervision, technical and business writing, and interviewing and hiring. My profiling showed that business development might be a great fit for me, so I decided to give it a shot. I competed with the editor of this book (Robbins-Roth) for a business development position at another biotech firm but ended up in the scientific affairs department at Syntex. I spent 2 years there, essentially getting an on-the-job, functional M.B.A.

Everything was done in teams, which put me in direct contact with people from all over Syntex. My title was senior medical researcher, and the job included acting as a technical liaison to the U.S. business and legal divisions; working on research communications, product management, and development; planning business strategies; assessing due diligence and technical assessment; doing competitive surveillance; and working on technical support and interpretation for product liability lawsuits. I had the opportunity to do some data analysis for clinical trials, and I managed the team developing a computerized information management system. I also published a paper on drug interactions with birth control medications that was detailed to OB/GYN doctors all over the world and worked with product managers and advertising.

While this was a wonderful chance to broaden my horizons and become proficient in a wide range of fields, it was a dead-end job because I did not have the M.B.A. then required to get into the business development department. By 1987, when my husband headed off to Europe on sabbatical, I took a year-long leave of absence from Syntex and joined him.

THE NEXT STEP: FINANCIAL CONSULTING

When I returned, I faced the decision to keep commuting from San Francisco to the same job, to go back to school for an M.B.A., or to come up with something completely different. And that is how I became an independent consultant for the next 10 years.

This mutation came via a consulting client, Bridgemere Capital. The people at Bridgemere taught me about finance and urged me to become an investment banker. While I loved the finance side, I realized that I didn't want to be a banker—I wanted to be an analyst who focused on biotech stocks.

Sadly, I could not get a job in San Francisco as an analyst at that time, mostly because my science and medicine knowledge exceeded that of the hiring managers in town. I headed for New York, the home base of most stock analysts, and started interviewing for jobs. The head of research at Dean Witter gave me very appealing advice—you don't need an M.B.A.; just go take corporate finance and securities analysis courses and then start publishing stock research reports on biotech companies. I took his advice and started a newsletter to show my potential market what I could do.

Mentors continued to be very important all along my career path. Another one was Dr. Carol Hall, a fellow scientist gone astray who became a banker and analyst before joining forces with the editor of this book. Carol taught me how to dress and how to understand the milieu; we both loved talking about finance.

It was now 1990. I was juggling work with being married to a professor and coping with his travel and commitments. I figured I would stay with the analyst work long enough to get trained and then I could make a good living as a financial consultant.

That year, I met another key mentor. Richard Bock, affectionately known as Biobock for his active support for biotech stocks, was pivotal in helping me build my business. He recruited subscribers for my newsletter and mailed copies to his clients. People liked what I wrote. I was one of the first to set up a useful format for reporting on biotech stocks based on cash, cash burn, and stratifying companies by product development status.

My newsletter led to my next job, in 1992 to 1993, with Soundview Financial Group. This firm wanted to build up a biotech analyst group, liked my analysis in the newsletter, and invited me to join their team. I knew I needed to spend time on Wall Street to really understand the stock market, and Soundview was willing to let me commute between San Francisco and their base in Connecticut. This job gave me a great chance to learn about the stock market and trading, and I got to meet institutional investors—the people with the big bucks to invest.

• •

"My newsletter led to my next job, in 1992 to 1993, with Soundview Financial Group."

• •

Sadly, the Soundview brokers weren't able to sell the biotech story to their existing customer base and could not understand my reports. Most biotech companies lacked the classic components by which investors measure stock performance—P/E ratios, earnings, and other such factors. My husband was about to found his second biomedical company, GeneMedicine, Inc., and I was getting tired of commuting. I came back home in 1993 and started Biobusiness Resources, Inc., an independent consulting company focused on portfolio assembly and assessment and technology assessment.

As time went by, I followed my interests and focused more on financial issues and less on business development. I became a registered investment advisor and started Szoka Capital Management in 1995. I already had my broker's license and continued to consult mostly for institutional investors.

Two things convinced me to change paths yet again. First, I tried to raise a "mixed use" investment fund. This began when I met a biochemist at Roche who became a mezzanine venture capitalist in the medical device arena. He convinced me to try to raise a $10 million fund, along with an ex-CFO of Amgen. The ex-CFO became a seed venture capitalist after he retired from the top finance slot at Amgen Corporation. We met when I followed Amgen as an analyst.

We spent 2 years trying to raise $10 million to invest in small capitalization public stocks, private investments in public equity transactions (PIPEs), and mezzanine venture rounds. It became clear that we were thinking far too small for the investors we were approaching—they wanted to hand out $100 million at a time to a team with a track record and to co-invest with other members of their "old boys network." If we had gone instead to wealthy individuals and foreign governments, we probably could have raised the fund. But when we reached the end of 2 years with no results, we decided to call it a day. It was January 1998, and I was job hunting again!

BACK TO ACADEMIA BUT NOT TO THE LAB!

At the big analyst meeting held in San Francisco every January, I ran into Dave Aston, head of a technology transfer licensing group at the University of California (UC) Office of Technology Transfer (OTT), located in the office of UC's president. I had first met Dave when I was a member of the board of directors of a biomedical start-up that had licensed its main technology from UC, a technology managed by Dave's group. I told him that with my daughter heading off to college, I was looking for a position. Dave told me about an opening for licensing officer in his group. I sent in a résumé and interviewed at OTT. While I certainly did not have the traditional career path to this job and did not know the details of patents and licensing, the company decided that with my science background, I was smart enough to figure it out. I had not worked for anyone else for 10 years and was not at all sure about this, but I was willing to give it a shot. This turned out to be a very smart bet.

The honeymoon period for this job was very short. I began on April Fools' Day in 1998; by August, a senior person left the office, and my caseload went from 60 to about 200. Then Dave left, and I ended up with about 400! I was still learning patent management and licensing, though deal negotiation flowed from my previous experience. Most problems arise from bad contracts. In the course of solving these problems, you learn a lot about the details of the process.

THE LIFE OF A LICENSING OFFICER

I spent 5 years in this new career and liked everything about technology transfer. It is tremendously interesting—you are managing science and coordinating with lawyers and scientists to create intellectual property (IP). You have to understand business to find the best home for the IP. The primary focus of my group included research tools, diagnostics, and therapeutics.

I loved this new job at the junction of science, business, and academia. It is never dull on any level: the science is very exciting, and dealing with the scientists, lawyers, and business people is a lot like herding cats. Patent strategy was especially interesting to me with my background in both business and finance. I was able to help the patent attorneys think about designing patent claims that would be commercially important, not just trying for the greatest number of claims. This concept of commercial relevance could be tough to get across to the professors, and I sometimes found myself trying to explain why great science was not always worth cold cash to companies.

This concept of commercial relevance being as important as scientific value is showing up more frequently in academic institutions that rely on large federal grants to support on-campus research. The University of California is only one institution that encourages faculty to be entrepreneurial.

A licensing officer follows an invention from cradle to grave. You do everything from getting that first disclosure from the academic researcher, deciding if it warrants a patent, and managing the patent process, which includes filing the application and handling office actions and interferences (when two different parties file the same invention with the patent office). I really enjoyed working on interferences, which are basically a form of litigation: two different parties file patents claiming the same invention. The patent office can't issue both patents. There can be only one inventor, and the patent is awarded to the person who made the invention first. You have to prove your case to the patent office, which is very complicated and very interesting.

During my time at UC, I was responsible for initiating a major litigation for breach of contract by one of our licensees. It was very complicated (auditing financial reports and plowing through pages of legalese) and risky because the original contract language was less than crystal clear. But we ended up with a settlement in the six-figure range, making it all worthwhile for UC, the University inventors, and the licensee.

Director of Technology Transfer: The Business of IP

After I reached my 5-year mark at UC, I realized that there was nowhere to go. I was in a senior position, well regarded, and felt that my performance should have rated an assistant director title. Sadly, the director of my office did not feel the same way. I kept applying for higher positions with UC and had great support from academics who had good experiences working with me, only to find that many of the positions are posted publicly when the office already has someone in mind for the job. After this happened three times, budget cuts hit the UC system. If I wanted to go up, I clearly would have to go out.

I was very fortunate to be offered my current position with University of Washington in Seattle. I had the experience and good productivity and reputation they were looking for, and I clicked with the people on campus. And this office had all the elements I was looking for in a director position: the money and infrastructure resources needed to succeed. Some universities won't provide the right support for their tech transfer groups, making it very difficult to perform the job of transferring discoveries and patented technologies from academics into companies for the public good.

It is a challenge to make the tech transfer office a profit center, and it definitely takes some time. First, you need to build up the patent portfolio, and then you need to find licensees to bring in the cash. Most companies that come sniffing around university tech transfer offices are simply signing confidential disclosure agreements (CDAs) just to see what you have so that they can try to design around those potential claims in their own labs. Licensees usually appear after patent claims have issued, and companies judge that they need the licensed rights to those claims to conduct their business.

Even when you do get licenses, it's tough to make net cash—to bring in more money than you spend on running the office. University patent licenses tend to come cheap. Most of the time, your team's patent claims represent only a subset of what the licensing company needs to practice the invention. The company often has to license technology from several other places before it can get a product into the marketplace, generating what is termed "stacking royalties." If the royalty fees are too expensive, the company can't see a path to profitability and often will drop the project and the attendant license.

A university tech transfer group also has to pay attention to the requirements imposed by the source of funding for the research. The National Institutes of Health, which funds much of the research handled by my group at University of Washington, has rules and guidelines covering inventions made with their grant funds. For example, there is a lot of pressure to make research tools available nonexclusively (thus more cheaply) to many licensees. Under the Bayh-Dole Act, which set up rules for government-funded tech transfer, universities are required to give precedence to small companies (usually not the highest bidder) and firms with substantial manufacturing in the United States.

You have to be aware of what the market will bear. In our sector, deals tend to include up-front fees under $1 million, a yearly maintenance fee, some milestone payments, and royalties, if a product is ever developed. Many licensed technologies never result in products or products producing six-figure royalty revenues. A director tries to fill the patent pipeline as best he or she can with inventions that will be commercially useful. Research tools are very common inventions coming out of university research: for example, UC had a lot of mouse models that became very frequently used by both academic and for-profit researchers. My business background helped us set up models for generating more revenue based on market value and availability of the research tools developed at UC. Once in a great while, you get a big producer—the Cohen/Boyer patent (covering the basic gene splicing technique of genetic engineering) was an excellent license for Stanford and UC. Its license was priced well, so everyone could afford to use it, and it still made millions of dollars for the universities.

People focus too much on the money aspect of the tech transfer office, when most of what we do is provide service. It's very possible to have 1000 patents and not make much revenue. The top patent producing schools, such as MIT, Stanford, Columbia, and UC, generate their big cash returns over a period of years. For most schools, you are doing a good job if you simply make enough on licenses to cover the costs to file all those patents. If you manage to generate enough cash to actually cover the full cost of running the office, that's great! In addition, public universities have an overlay of state law and policy that limit flexibility in some situations, and academic freedom issues are very important to consider. So doing technology transfer in an academic setting is complicated and challenging.

A Typical Day as Director

Basically, I am in meetings all day, jumping from topic to topic. I am responsible for four different groups, 25 people altogether: (i) licensing managers; (ii) a patent management group; (iii) a legal affairs group that handles lawsuits, interferences, contract issues, structure and function of our database, and required federal reporting; (iv) the Material Transfer Agreement group that handles 500 to 600 MTAs each year.

UW TechTransfer has four groups altogether: Invention Licensing (my group, about half the office); Digital Ventures, which is responsible for copyright, software, and database management; Finance & Business Operations; and Policy & Strategic Initiatives. We all report to the vice provost of intellectual property and technology transfer. Our entire group is very large for a university tech transfer operation and is about half the size of the central tech transfer group for the University of California.

It is quite demanding, having so many people in four different groups all looking to me for direction! In addition to all the team meetings, I have been working with individuals in the group on licensing issues, goals and priorities of the department, and how to triage. Once they understand our goals, I use frequent one-on-one meetings to give direction and then back off and let them do their jobs.

I meet regularly with my boss, the vice provost. We meet formally every Monday morning, talk almost daily when he is in town, and use e-mail to stay in touch outside of office hours. Because I work so closely with him,

I am very lucky that he is a wonderful leader, a good politician, and has a work style that fits well with mine.

Luckily, all my experience to date prepared me very well for this potential chaos. I am able to solve problems and direct people on how to solve their issues. I was brought in to help reorganize and focus the office, with stronger business and management ethics. My boss set out the road map, and my job is to make it happen.

I have spent a significant amount of time in this early stage of my new job figuring out the turf by meeting with deans, department chairs, and the major inventors on campus. They all want to know the status of our IP portfolio and whether we are generating big licensing fees. A big part of my job is supporting these groups in their goals and educating the faculty about IP, while supporting the creation of IP that can be helpful to them and the campus.

Meeting with the inventors is crucial. You must understand how the IP fits into the long-term strategy for their lab, which tends to be focused on getting papers published and grants funded. I believe it is important to get the inventors excited about seeing their work put to use in the outside world and to engage them in the process.

The faculty here is learning more about the IP process and about the pros and cons of putting inventions into this format. I want them talking to my office early in the process so that I can understand how they want their technology used. It is crucial to be sure that the IP process does not interfere with their grant applications and that the inventors' plans for building their own companies don't get them into a conflict of interest.

It is very common for universities and those companies wanting to license our technology to have goals and objectives in direct conflict. Companies like to structure deals that include sponsored research, that allow them to own everything coming out of the sponsored lab, and that enable them to use money to get the terms they want. The tech transfer office can find itself taking the blame for holding up licensing deals when the problem is actually in the company.

You have to be clever enough to smoke out the real situation, which often allows it to be resolved quickly. I have found that my experience on Wall Street, especially learning the due diligence process, was wonderful training for this!

My schedule is very hectic, and there is no routine day other than the fact that they all include many meetings, a lot of emails, and many late nights. Typically, from 8:00 to 11:00 A.M., I have meetings with my boss and fellow directors, answer e-mail, and work on reports and situations. From 11:00 A.M. on, I meet with my staff, address our mandate to help facility start-ups (which includes meeting with potential investors), solve problems, direct traffic, and put out fires. My goal: after I have been here for a year, I expect things to be running more smoothly, have more tasks delegated, and hopefully have more free time!

Pros and Cons of the Job

My favorite thing about the job: everything! It has been very satisfying to take a situation that was in trouble and turn unhappy people into happy, productive people. I enjoy finding the "win-win" in the situation and creating the IP asset. I actually like the "herding cats" aspect of getting all these diverse groups to work together and developing something tangible out of it. I love that the topics covered by this job are so diverse: I still love research and science, but I don't actually want to do the experiments. Through this job, I get a very broad view of what is happening in science through a meshing of computer technology and biology, new plants, cool tools, and so on. I was feeling pigeonholed at UC, and now I have wildly diverse teams of people and inventors to work with—it is NOT dull!

> *"I actually like the "herding cats" aspect of getting all these diverse groups to work together and developing something tangible out of it."*

My least favorite part of the job: when the IP office gets blamed unfairly for why something isn't working out. I have found that many companies get frustrated with universities because they just don't understand the basic concepts of the university's obligations to its faculty and students and to the public. Some of our obligations are determined by law! Companies often expect to get the same kinds of terms that they get from other companies. We find ourselves in the same arguments all the time. The key is to avoid losing your temper and also look for ways to gently educate companies about the university obligations via Web sites and talks.

Ultimately, the pay scales are low compared to what you get paid in industry. Because I was productive at UC, my pay went from being terrible to pretty good. Tech transfer offices are getting more competitive with industry, especially as they increasingly recruit staff from industry.

Where can you grow in this career track? You can probably make it to vice provost if you want to stay in academia. Another path for university licensing officers is to head into the business development in industry or to become a patent agent or patent attorney.

Personality traits that are very helpful in this job include the ability to manage stress and to triage what you are doing, to conduct thorough due diligence, to mediate disputes, and to find the facts hidden in strong rhetoric. This job is very people intensive, and you MUST have good skills for dealing with difficult people. You must love the science and be able to get excited about it. You must want to learn new things all the time.

This is a bad job if you don't like working with many different types of people and can't handle stress. You will always have more work to do than is possible, and you will need to prioritize, organize, and have good time management skills. You have to be able to compromise, although there are some points where you have to walk away from a negotiation. I have found that as long as you are communicating openly and are able to show progress, the professors take the disappointments pretty well.

How to Find These Jobs

To find out about these jobs, check out the following organizations:

- The Association of University Technology Managers (www.autm.net), which describes itself as "a nonprofit organization with membership of more than 3200 technology managers and business executives who manage IP. AUTM's members represent more than 300 universities, research institutes, teaching hospitals, and a similar number of companies and government organizations."
- The Licensing Executive Society (www.les.org) is, according to their site, "a professional society comprised of more than 5000 members engaged in the transfer, use, development, manufacture, and marketing of IP. The LES membership includes a wide range of professionals, including business executives, lawyers, licensing consultants, engineers, academicians, scientists, and government officials."

Almost everyone relevant belongs to these organizations. Look at AUTM and LES sites for meetings, networking, and job listings. I found my latest job on one of these sites!

How to Get the Job

Very few people come to a tech transfer job with all the skills needed. Most of us are middle-aged and have had several other jobs and have found our way to tech transfer based on our growing skills and love of science.

Start by doing bench research in a small company; network with the IP people at the company and go from there. An M.B.A. can be useful, but I would rather hire people who did applied science and learned something about companies, and then I could teach them the rest. Ethical standards are high. If you want to remain focused on one area, stay in a company rather than heading for an academic post. Some experience in finance can be helpful, but being in the trenches in a company and taking a research project and trying to move it to commercialization is wonderful experience.

PROVIDING SERVICES TO COMPANIES

17

··········

CORPORATE

COMMUNICATIONS:

Helping Companies Sell Their Stories

●●●●●●●●●●●●●●●●

Tony Russo, Ph.D.

Cofounder and CEO of Noonan Russo

Often, lab scientists tell me that they love science, but they are tired of working in the lab. How can they work as scientists without having to work in a lab? How can they communicate the science without being the ones conducting it? One great answer is to enter the public relations (PR) field, working with technology-based clients.

About 10 years ago, it was unusual for recruiters in the PR profession to receive résumés from scientists, much less from those with Ph.D.s. After 8-plus years of advanced study, why would someone switch to a profession in which the typical participant has only a college degree? I have spent more than two decades as one of the few with a Ph.D. in PR, feeling like a misfit in a profession dominated by people with undergraduate degrees in English and journalism.

Suddenly, the climate has changed. I receive résumés from several applicants with Ph.D.s each week. Today, people seem more inclined to investigate alternative careers and move into professions that don't appear to directly use their graduate degrees.

For me, the realization that I could consider an alternative to further work in the field of psychology came when I was studying and conducting research at Harvard University. I saw my colleagues struggling to obtain even an entry-level job in a profession where they had spent 5 or more years studying at the advanced levels. These were bright people with a string of publications to their credit and short-term expectations no grander than landing a temporary adjunct professorship at a mid-tier state-run school.

My own hope of supporting myself with government research grants was cut short by the budding trend toward cost-cutting at the federal and state levels. And so, my entry into PR occurred not by design but rather by the need for employment. In fact, when I received my Ph.D., I hardly knew the PR profession existed.

I found the route to a PR career during a 2-year stint on Wall Street. I certainly wasn't the only one with a Ph.D. (or degree holder of any level, for that matter) to be tempted by Wall Street in the early 1980s. We all thought that Wall Street might be an interesting alternative to research (to say nothing of the money you could make, significantly more than as a post-doc). None of us had much in the way of direct qualifications for being on Wall Street. The common wisdom was "if I can get a Ph.D., then surely I can do a spreadsheet." Besides, there were a few role models successfully practicing on Wall Street, many from among my group at Harvard. Why not practice along with them?

My personal role model was a practicing psychiatrist from Yale who headed up a major bullion trading company. Why did he leave psychiatry? He was fond of telling me, "How much money could I have made in an hour, $100? In private practice you are limited by the amount of time you can work. In business you don't have those limitations."

Although money was not my motivation, my role model's ability to switch professions, for whatever reason, made me realize that I, who had invested less academic time in my pursuits, might qualify for a career change consideration. Role models become important in switching professions because they give you a yardstick to measure yourself against. In academia or in the lab, you simply look at your colleague across the hall. In PR, the only ways that you find out about others' academic training is through asking and being mentored. After a couple of years in what I now consider to be my second graduate degree, I found myself enjoying writing, research, and organization, three skills I needed to get my Ph.D. and three skills that are critical for success in PR. The pay was poor at that point and not what I had fantasized—around $12,500 per year, not nearly enough to survive in New York City! But I liked the work, and I was learning.

My first real introduction to PR was an undergraduate night course I took while I was on Wall Street. I applied what I learned in the course to my Wall Street job and quickly realized I had found my calling. I could research companies, learn about a lot of different professions, write, and organize. PR turned out to be a profession that was stimulating, interesting, and that had job openings! For me, the ability to later work alongside the health care profession, the very profession I had trained to become a member of, was an added incentive to make this move.

The professor of the PR course took me aside one evening and said I was wasting my time by working at a single private company and that to grow and develop in the field, I should work for a PR agency for at least 5 years. This would allow me to gain a variety of experiences working on several different accounts. She said I had talent but that I really needed further exposure, and she offered to point me in the right direction and write a letter of reference.

I took her advice and began to apply for jobs in the financial PR field. Remember, I was coming from Wall Street, and there were basically two specialties in PR: financial and general interest. At least I had a little experience to become a specialist!

I ended up at a small entrepreneurial financial PR firm that specialized in international companies. There we represented foreign companies doing business in the United States. It was a specialty that was being pioneered by the head of the agency.

Within 2 years, I saw this tiny agency grow to have offices in London, Brussels, Sydney, Hong Kong, and Tokyo. The rapid growth was a result of the leadership of the young CEO and the fact that the company had established a niche market. So, I learned lesson number one—put together a unique niche strategy that requires fairly high barriers to entry (in this case, it was knowledge of world capital markets), specialize, then aggressively establish yourself in the field. With that important lesson learned, I moved on to gain more experience at other agencies.

I seemed to end up at agencies that were young, entrepreneurial, and in niche market areas. The agencies were all growing rapidly. Now there were more specialties such as real estate, health care, entertainment, and so on. I tried my hand at real estate, then at health care. By this time I had developed a real skill—I was good at organizing, and I seemed to have a knack for understanding the media, its needs, concerns, and politics. Also, I was good at putting a story together—seeing news when perhaps others did not and, more importantly, knowing when a story was not newsworthy or what elements it would need to become newsworthy.

But health care excited me. I was deeply interested in research, and to have the ability to understand it, synthesize it, and place it in a broader context was a challenge. I had spent several years studying medical psychology at Columbia University and at Johns Hopkins, and maybe now I could use some of that training in this new area of specialty. Maybe my life was coming full circle.

Then biotechnology was born. I had the good fortune to be working for an agency that had a biotech account (those were the days when there were only a handful of biotech companies). I began to pioneer a new area of PR: health care and biotech.

Success came quickly. I loved the work, I knew what I was talking about, and I quickly became one of the few experts in the field.

It was at that point that opportunity struck. My colleague across the hall asked me if I might be interested in striking out—building a new firm with her. I realized that I had all the ingredients I needed to be successful: skill, knowledge of medicine, and schooling in entrepreneurship from my previous positions. It was the beginning of the biotech movement, and I was in the right place at the right time.

Noonan Russo, now a division of Euro RSCG Life RP, quickly established itself as a leading firm in this area. We were specialists, and we circulated in the biotech and health care industries. And now nearly 17 years later, I have candidates for jobs, not unlike myself, sending me résumés.

So, what are the steps to break into the communications business, now that we with Ph.D.s don't have to be pioneers anymore?

MAKING THE MOVE

Many people with Ph.D.s who now come through my door at Noonan Russo looking for jobs and advice are not as fortunate as the undergraduates I see who knew from their freshman years that they wanted to work in PR and who have methodically sought out PR internships each summer. The candidates with Ph.D.s are smart, but they are largely uncertain about what they would like to do with their life outside of the lab. As people who have attained the highest academic degree possible, they usually have a strong sense of ego and are accustomed to working independently. This can make it tough to make the shift to working as part of a team, alongside people with more direct experience but fewer academic accolades.

All of our clients are businesses related to the biomedical field. This means that our employees need to understand the technical implications of the products and services we are presenting to the press and investors, and they also need communication skills. I often have to choose between an applicant with a strong PR background and someone who has a good technical background in the biosciences but lacks the essential PR skills needed to be successful in an agency setting.

• •
"In my business, a person must know how to write a news release and how to write for a nonscientific audience, as well as how to construct and write a PR program."
• •

In my business, a person must know how to write a news release and how to write for a nonscientific audience, as well as how to construct and write a PR program. That person must also have a basic understanding of chemistry and biology and must feel comfortable in communicating with the Wall Street community. It is a large skill set and one that few applicants have when they interview for an entry-level position with an agency such as Noonan Russo. Whether these skills are acquired on the job, in school, or through natural talents makes selecting the "right" candidates difficult.

So for me, there is always a gamble that the people I hire will be motivated to acquire the skills they don't have and use their current skills to add value to our organization. People with Ph.D.s almost have to forget that they have an advanced degree because they must learn a new set of skills to work in an environment where many may be threatened by their academic training. At Noonan Russo, we divide our staff into several groups: those who are interested in the investment community (investor relations), those who want to work with the press (media relations), those who like to write (corporate communications), and those who are interested in marketing (product communications). Each group requires a different set of skills and a different way of viewing the world. For example, the following subsections provide a sample of some of the questions members of our interviewing team might ask.

Media Relations

To join the media group at Noonan Russo, we require a basic knowledge of the working media. This means that you must understand the answers to the following questions:

- What are the major publications important for client coverage, and why are they important?
- How do you write a news release, and what goes into the lead paragraph, the first paragraph, the second paragraph, and the boilerplate?
- What is an advance and an embargo? When do you move news? What are the laws regarding public disclosure? What is the difference between not for attribution, off the record, and on the record? What is news?
- Who are the important reporters for the different sectors, and what are they writing about? When do you call a reporter? What do you say? What do you say to a reporter who doesn't want to be bothered talking to you? What if the reporter hates talking to PR firms (learn not to flinch at the word "hack")?

Investor Relations

Two of the most critical issues for any company are how to raise financing and how to keep shareholders happy. A strong IR group can make a significant difference in a company's long-term success. Here, the importance of knowing how Wall Street operates is critical:

- What is the difference between a balance sheet and an income statement? What is a burn rate?
- Who are the major analysts that cover biotech, and which companies (your client? your client's competition?) do they write about?
- What are the major investment banks that finance in your client's sector?
- What are the leading companies in your client's sector? What are their products that might compete with your client's? How are they viewed compared with your client?
- What is the difference between the buy-side and the sell-side? What is the difference between retail and institutional investors?
- What are the trends driving the financial markets?
- What are the SEC regulations covering disclosure? What is the "quiet period"?
- What is Regulation FD?
- What is the Sarbans Oxley?

Product Communications

In the biomedical arena, product news is critical to a company's stock price, which in turn drives the company's ability to raise future financings and its ability to complete product research and development. Helping clients communicate clearly and in a timely fashion about their products in development is an important role. Some of the key issues include:

- What are the FDA rules regarding clinical trial result disclosures?
- What are the steps to FDA approval?
- What are the FDA advisory panels? How do they work?
- What is the difference between a PLA, a 510K, and an NDA?
- How do you launch a product? What are you allowed to say about the product and its competition? What isn't allowed? FDA regulations about disclosure can sometimes interfere with SEC disclosure requirements.

Corporate Communications

To keep shareholders on board and to gain new shareholders (as well as to fulfill SEC requirements), companies must maintain an ongoing stream of communication with the outside world. Some of the important issues for a PR firm working with such a company are indicated by the following questions:

- What are key corporate messages? This can be amazingly difficult for a company to verbalize, but it is critical, especially in a sector where there are 250 other companies competing for the attention of the press, Wall Street, and investors.
- How are these corporate messages best expressed to different audiences?
- What are the best tools to use: broadcast, Internet, print, or others?
- What are the elements of good corporate design, and why is it important?
- What makes a good corporate identity?
- How do you judge the right style of design to use and other such factors?

Naturally, we look not only at how well one can answer the above questions, but also at the candidate's portfolio of existing work. How have the job candidates demonstrated that they can perform the above tasks? What is the quality of their previous work? How can their references support their candidacy?

HOW DO I BREAK INTO THE PROFESSION IF I DON'T HAVE THESE SKILLS?

Get some PR experience: work as a volunteer, take PR courses, or try to get an internship at a firm. Imagine that you are still in graduate school. Don't focus on a salary; just get the experience so that you can demonstrate to a prospective employer that you want to be in PR and that you have enough skills to be able to be productive from the first day of work. It is perhaps the most difficult job you will ever try to get because few organizations want to serve as a training ground for someone who has little working knowledge of his or her profession—or even worse, for someone who is unsure of what they want to do in life.

YOU HAVE THE JOB! NOW WHAT CAN YOU EXPECT?

The best employees we have had are always the ones who can't seem to learn enough, who are continually curious. PR, unlike other professions, is a bit unstructured. Anything can happen at any moment. The stock market can take a dive, a product can fail in clinical trials, and a researcher can commit fraud. And it is the PR professional who will be called upon for advice and quick action. One needs to be organized, calm, efficient, and able to attend to details for multiple clients, usually simultaneously.

So what is a typical day like? It can begin with a news release, or several news releases, which can mean getting up in time to distribute the release as early as 3:00 A.M. Remember, some firms operate on European time. When it is 8:30 A.M. in Europe, it is 2:30 A.M. in New York. Sending a news release might involve e-mailing it to a group of publications you have chosen to get that news. This group may vary, depending on the news you are distributing. For example, a science discovery would go to a different group of reporters and interested individuals than would a personnel announcement. Besides going to a different list of publications, the news might go to different reporters at the same publication.

Once you have sent out the news release, it is time to follow-up with the group of reporters to whom you have sent it. Are they interested in the story, and will they report it? Was there an interesting aspect of the announcement that they may have missed? Why was the paper so important? What role does the research play within the current body of research on the topic? In short, why is the paper important and deserving of coverage? Although many of these questions may have been answered in the news release, the role of the PR professional is to illuminate, to help educate the reporter about your client, to provide access to your client, to answer the reporter's questions, and to make recommendations regarding with whom the reporter might speak at the company.

If you work in the investor relations area, you might call a Wall Street analyst or a mutual fund manager about the news, particularly if the announcement was made by a public company. If that person were convinced that the news was significant, the analyst might issue an internal note to her firm about the announcement, and perhaps she might recommend purchase of the stock. She might also issue an external report supporting the same conclusion. If she is a fund manager, she might purchase the stock.

But what if the announcement is negative? What if a clinical trial has failed? To be prepared for negative news, or crisis management as it is called in the PR business, is a critical component of PR. Develop a plan—before it happens, understand your different audiences, what their needs might be, and how to provide them with timely information. Your audience might be the company's employees, its shareholders, those who write about and follow the company, community officials, and so on. The message might be different for each audience. And while the temptation might be to put a positive spin on the announcement, one of the most important roles of the PR professional is to get the news out quickly and accurately.

In addition to the news that drives your day, a PR professional might write a brochure, devise a PR program or communications strategy, write a slide show for the investment community, or prepare a client for a meeting with the press or with the financial community. Your day could include speaker training, media training, or writing and producing a video. It could also involve finding a name for a new company, renaming an old one, or helping to create a corporate identity or logo.

In terms of a skill set, the PR field can allow you to use your creative skills, your writing skills, your scientific knowledge, your knowledge of the biotech field, and so on. It is a field so varied, requiring so many different types of skills, that it is nearly impossible to be perfectly trained before entering the field.

Salary and Job Titles

Entry-level positions start at around $35,000 for most large urban centers. A hard-working employee can expect to advance from this level within a year of starting the job. At the vice president level, the salary will be range between $100,000 and $150,000.

At most agencies, progress is measured by client satisfaction, the ability to generate new business, and talent—producing creative work. Because PR involves a lot of juggling, you must maintain an air of calm at all times. The ability to multitask is important, and you must do this while paying attention to the many details inherent in the position. As you advance, you become responsible for larger accounts with bigger budgets and with increasingly sophisticated communications programs.

The alternative to working at a PR agency is to work in-house at a pharmaceutical or biotech company. An in-house position may have many of the same responsibilities as does a position at an external PR agency. The job might involve responsibility for internal communications or product communications (e.g., news releases, communications with the media, etc.) with a greater emphasis on helping to position the story so that the PR agency can take it to a wider audience. The internal tasks might be divided into investor relations responsibilities and media or corporate communications responsibilities. Tasks such as writing might fall to the in-house person.

In smaller companies, you may need to be cross-functional. In larger organizations, an internal communications position might exist. Public affairs, crisis management, and governmental relations may also fall into the realm of the communications group. A large pharmaceutical company might employ 60 people in the communications area. The main difference, however, between an agency position and one in-house is that at an agency, a person usually works with many clients on a number of projects. As a result, the in-house person often has a greater understanding of the company that he or she is working for than might an outside person.

In an agency, most newcomers begin as an account coordinator or junior account executive. If the candidate has experience in the communications business, it might be possible to begin as an account executive or senior account executive. In a biotech or other small corporation, one might begin as a manager of communications or as a writer.

Regardless of the position, you might take a pay cut if you are coming from academia. When I started in the business, I was told, "Your Ph.D. doesn't matter to us; you have to start at the same level as everyone else." So my first few years were viewed as further graduate training. It is important to focus on what you learn in the first few years and not on the salary. If you are good, your scientific training will give you the push you need to move up the career ladder to the assistant vice-president and vice-president level.

Training

Training in PR is a daily activity. There are few formal courses that you can take. Until recently, few schools even offered courses. Now you can get accreditation in PR and can even be licensed by the Public Relations Society of America (PRSA), the trade group governing the field. To become licensed, you must work in the PR field full-time for 5 years and must pass rigorous written and oral exams. Because the accreditation was introduced in 1964, and because the industry has historically not pushed accreditation, few professionals are certified. Although the PRSA has made great efforts to license people in the profession, this has little impact on your ability to land a job or an account. However, if you want to rise in the PRSA hierarchy, licensing is critical.

But what if you have not had any formal courses, and you are fresh out of a doctoral program? How long will it take for you to gain a working knowledge of the field? The answer is about 2 years. In that time, you may write and distribute many news releases, annual reports, and brochures. You may produce slide presentations, set up analyst meetings, and perhaps organize media tours or investor road shows. You will work on Web sites, navigate through a crisis or two, and write many PR programs. The result is a feeling of confidence that you will be able to manage most PR tasks. As you advance through the hierarchy, you will be able to handle more and more responsibilities. The more experience you have, the better you will be able to advise a client.

Mobility

It has often been said that working for an agency is a critical professional move in a PR career because it gives you a wide variety of experiences that will help you make more educated judgments. The skills and experiences gained from working in an agency will be useful in almost any PR setting. Working for clients on different programs in various situations gives you a wide range of life experiences (and great juggling skills). In-house, there is less variety, and the focus may be on just one product. This is the difference between being a generalist and being a specialist.

As a specialist, you might work only with the media on biotech accounts. As a generalist, you might work on investor relations, media relations, or annual reports for a variety of firms that range from financial service companies to entertainment companies. It is like the difference between being a liberal arts major in college and choosing a major for an advanced degree. While larger PR agencies prefer generalists, the smaller, boutique agencies and the corporations prefer the specialist. To become a specialist will make you very employable in a single profession. If there are few jobs in that field, however, you might have fewer options.

As a person with a Ph.D., you will find it easier to get a job as a specialist because you have a specific area of expertise that few other people have in PR. In fact, this is your key selling point. If you have a Ph.D., you probably enjoy the field you have specialized in, and you want to stay close to the profession.

WHERE DO I GO TO FIND OUT ABOUT PR?

Many directories can inform you about PR companies and their specialty. The most famous of these is *O'Dwyer's Directory of Public Relations Firms*. It contains a directory of all United States agencies and their specialties. It also contains a listing of their clients. Conversely, you can look up the clients you might like to work with and find out who represents them. The names of the appropriate contacts, vice presidents, and other relevant individuals are listed, as well as phone numbers, addresses, and listings of branch offices. This directory can be obtained in the career center of most libraries. The PRSA in New York City has a large research library that can be used for a fee. You can also purchase it on the Web.

O'Dwyer's also publishes a directory that lists communication officers in major American companies. This directory can give you a feel for the type of communications program a company has—how many people are employed in the department, who is the contact person, and so on.

How Do I Prepare for a Job Interview?

It is important to do your research before the job interview. Make sure you view the company's Web site and that you have a keen sense of the company's mission and its direction. Try to find out as much as you can about the company—read the annual report, look at brochures, try to learn if it has won any awards, and look up the background of the person who is interviewing you. Is the company listed in *Who's Who*? Has it received any awards? What is its reputation? Has anyone written about the company? You might also want to conduct a Google search. This is a computer database search that allows you to view articles written about a person, company, or subject.

The only way to show a potential employer that you are serious about a communications job is to demonstrate your breadth of knowledge about the PR field and the specific knowledge you have about the company—its communications strategy as you see it. That, and establishing good rapport, will likely land you a second interview and possibly even a job offer.

Remember, your goal is to get your foot in the door and to find a job that will allow you to learn as much as possible. Be persistent. One candidate with a Ph.D. recently got a job with us only after numerous interviews. He maintained that he could learn PR and that he was so motivated that he would start at any salary at any level. He had researched the profession, and he had spoken with a number of headhunters in the field, whom he identified through newspaper ads, and he narrowed his search to one agency. With that kind of sales pitch, we had to hire him.

● ●
"Remember, your goal is to get your foot in the door and to find a job that will allow you to learn as much as possible."
● ●

The Personality Profile

To be successful in communications, it helps to be an extrovert. Type B personalities—the calmer personalities—are better suited for this profession. Remember, you will find yourself in many crisis situations in which you will have to maintain a calm attitude. On the agency side, there is a crisis at every turn, and the ability to maintain one's cool while attending to the many details of a difficult situation is a personality trait that the job demands.

The profile is slightly different when you are in-house. It represents the opportunity to learn a lot about a single company—to fully understand the drug development process, to be a spokesperson for the organization. While you may not have to attend to the volume of potential crisis work, you have to be able to navigate through the corporate structure. Your job and your responsibilities may have a greater likelihood of change as the organization evolves. A drug that is not approved by the FDA can have a severe impact on job viability in the PR area, which is often viewed as the most expendable department in a company.

To deal with this type of change, you need to be flexible and to look for opportunities in an organization where you can add value during crises to help a company rebuild. PR requires a number of skills, many of which can't be learned. You need to be extroverted, gregarious, personable, decisive, and a good and quick writer, and you must demonstrate confidence and a sense of control. While other skills are helpful (including knowledge of the industry, business acumen, and knowledge of science), personality and persona count enormously.

Unlike lab work, where you often work in isolation, PR is a group-oriented profession. In an agency, there may be many individuals focused on different areas. The "gestalt" requires interaction among the group— brainstorming, sending proposals to the client, and distributing actions among the group. You seldom work in isolation.

A corporate setting may have similar strictures, and a hierarchy of approvals may be required before action is taken. In smaller companies, you are able to go directly to the president with a proposal.

DIFFICULTIES AND PLEASURES

Stressful is a word that is used frequently to describe PR work, and for good reason. It is very stressful to balance so many projects at different levels and to attend to so many details simultaneously, especially knowing that one dropped ball can cause incredible chaos. These situations can take their toll on you.

In an agency, each client thinks he or she is your only client. Crises always occur at the worst possible time. Disaster at Chernobyl happened at 1:23 A.M., the Three Mile Island incident occurred just after 4:00 A.M., and the Exxon Valdez accident happened shortly after midnight. A client does not care that you might have five other news releases to send, all of which are very important to other clients. The Food and Drug Administration does not consult with you about when they will approve—or reject—a product.

But if you can manage and if you like a challenge, PR gives you great opportunity for creativity. Unlike the lab where there is a procedure for everything, PR is an open universe. There is no science. There are precedents, but few hard and fast rules. It gives you great latitude and the chance to try new ways of doing things. While

• •
"Unlike the lab where there is a procedure for everything, PR is an open universe. There is no science."
• •

there may be certain formats, certain ways of writing, PR is in no way as rigorous as science. In fact, creativity is at a premium in PR positions. The best professionals are the ones who are the most creative.

But what is creativity? Many people imagine that PR is like advertising. People get together and dream up an ad campaign and brainstorm lots of ideas. In PR, the ability to have this sort of brainstorming session can be limited. Creativity in PR is the ability to help maneuver clients out of difficult situations: a drug fails in clinical trials; a CEO resigns; a competitor releases a study that questions the viability of your drug; or, on the positive side, your client just got published in *Nature*, so you need to decide what to do. There is a limited number of options, and you have to consider that you might have to deal with the Securities and Exchange Commission or with FDA regulations. Within these guidelines, however, there is room to deal creatively with various audiences: the general public, investors, physicians, the scientific community, and others.

WHERE CAN I FIND A PR JOB?

One of the best places to find a job these days is on the Internet. There are many jobs listed on Job Trak and on other university postings. In addition, some PR agencies, such as Noonan Russo, biotech, and pharmaceutical firms, also post jobs on their home pages.

Still, the best way to find a job is to do a little research. Look through the O'Dwyer's listing of PR and communications positions in the library. Do as much research as possible, and then send a pitch letter to the firm in which you are interested. Be specific about why you want to work there. Why are you interested in the firm? Why does your background make you a good fit?

Another way to find a job is through the old network system. Attend some of the investor conferences. Get to know people in the industry. Perhaps you could visit with companies and inquire as to what type of skills they require. Then you could build up your résumé, either through course work or as a volunteer.

Finally, you could read the classifieds in major newspapers such as the *New York Times* and the *Wall Street Journal*. The PRSA local chapters also post jobs in their state newsletters, as does O'Dwyer's PR/Marketing Communications Web site. Information on all these publications is available through the PRSA.

And be persistent!

18
· · · · · · · · · ·

EXECUTIVE SEARCH:

The Hunt for Exceptional Talent

· · · · · · · · · · · · · · · · ·

Bente Hansen, Ph.D.
Founder, Bente Hansen & Associates

I didn't set out to be a headhunter when I pursued my advanced degree. My entry into the workforce was as a college associate professor teaching anatomy and physiology.

Why and how did I make this transition? My career has taken many turns and has included a few high-risk entrepreneurial positions, but I have maximized my experiences to enhance my skill set. Experiences such as doing business development and marketing and sales, writing business plans, writing Small Business Innovation Research (SBIR) grants, starting my own company (Medical Impact), and running a preventive medicine center have helped me prepare for a career that I am committed to and am passionate about—retained executive search.

My transition was not a direct one. I found out about this industry first from people working for executive search firms that contacted me regarding opportunities they had available. Pay attention if you receive such calls! They are directed to you because the recruiter has researched you as a possible candidate for a prospective job or as a source of recommendations.

I was curious about the recruiting industry because it seemed like a business with great growth potential, so I started asking questions of the recruiters contacting me. Most search professionals are personable and polite on the telephone. My next step was to meet with someone who was successful in the industry so that I could learn about and better appreciate the day-to-day schedule of an executive recruiter. I was introduced to a highly successful recruiter who owned her own practice and who has made a name for herself in the recruitment of engineers. She was kind enough to give me a tremendous amount of information and support.

I was truly at a crossroads in my career at the time. After introspection and conversations with peers and friends, I realized that my strengths were in my knowledge of science and health care, in business development, and in my direct experience in knowing the difference a leader can make in an organization. I also had a long-term goal of building my own company.

I did extensive due diligence on the industry and found that there were few books or related articles on this industry. With *effort*, I obtained some career books including articles written years ago. A book, *Career Makers*, included brief biographical summaries of top national recruiters and gave tremendous insight into the qualities that made these folks so successful.

Becoming a Recruiter

After gaining valuable experience and moving up to managing director positions at two major search firms, DHR International and Gilbert Tweed, I started Bente Hansen & Associates with a colleague. Our primary goals are as follows.

- To obtain search contracts with companies in the bioscience and technology sectors for the recruitment of senior management and board members on a retained basis
- To work in partnership with senior management to strategize regarding human capital issues and to attract the best person for the position, with regard to experience, skills, and cultural fit
- To differentiate this company from other well-known retained search firms by providing high quality service

Responsibilities and Attributes

There are three traditional positions in the search industry: researcher, associate, and consultant. Researchers typically identify candidates and have a wealth of resources at their disposal. Associates work on the telephone, qualifying candidates who have been identified. Consultants manage client relationships, interview candidates, and develop business. For bioscience and pharmaceutical searches, a person's knowledge of science is very important.

The Researcher

A researcher has the responsibility of using the computer, library, databases, directories, contacts, and other resources to gain information about companies and people who are on the company's target list. The Internet has become an invaluable resource. Keep in mind that, in most cases, companies are looking to bring in a candidate with a wealth of experience in their industry, so information about competitors is crucial. The researcher does not come face to face with the client or candidates.

These are the skills needed for a research position:

- Tactical knowledge of research
- Innovation and creativity
- Great computer skills
- Project management skills
- Knowledge of databases and search sites
- Ability to listen

The Associate

The associate's primary partner is the telephone, which he or she uses to identify, screen, and qualify candidates. Since the associate will be working on multiple assignments, project management skills and a thorough understanding of the company are important. The following is a breakdown of the traits needed for this role.

Skills needed for the associate level:

- Knowledge of the company and requirements of the position
- Knowledge of a variety of management positions and their functions
- Ability to differentiate clients from competitors
- Good listening skills
- Good communication skills
- Sales capability

- Ability to enjoy phone conversations
- Interest in person-to-person interactions
- Ability to prioritize
- Project management skills

The Consultant

The consultant manages the client relationship and has frequent face-to-face conversations with the client in addition to meetings with final candidates. This person would move to managing director or business owner as a next step.

Skills needed for the consultant position include the following:

- An ability to write and summarize scientific and technical information in layperson's terms
- Knowledge of scientific principles
- The objective/analytical ability to evaluate needs of clients
- Confidence in making presentations to upper management and boards of directors
- Ability to comprehend and communicate information about numerous companies
- Ability to manage time as an independent contractor and to juggle a multitude of projects that are at different stages of development
- Ability to provide quality service
- Ability to analyze the culture of a company and to find candidates who are the best fit
- Ability to obtain information from potential candidates
- Good project management of time and resources
- Ability to work with many different types of people, from the CEO to director of biology to the vice president of manufacturing
- Ability to be a good salesperson (the company will compete with many others for the best candidate)
- Interest in taking risks (some of the fee could come from equity)
- Sharp assessment skills
- Knowledge of industry trends

- Ability to lead a research team
- Ability to create a network

It is very important that you enjoy meeting new people and that you have the ability to maintain your existing network of contacts. This network is critical to identifying strong candidates for your clients and for finding new clients. If you are shy or have difficulty asking questions of people you don't know well, this may not be the job for you.

It is important to be a self-starter—in most cases, nobody is going to call you with the candidates; you are going to have to be proactive in tracking them down. You need to have the interest and curiosity to learn about people, new technologies, and new companies in the industry you serve. Without that, you will limit your ability to understand your clients because you will not really understand their business and the issues that drive that business.

You have to be proficient at project management, and you have to be able to track and monitor multiple searches while meeting key deadlines. In most cases, you will be juggling several client projects simultaneously, and all of those clients will expect you to stay on top of their project. Every delay they face in bringing the best person on board impacts their company's ability to meet its own milestones. This means that you must be flexible in your work hours to accommodate clients and candidates on the east coast and west coast, as well as internationally. You can often speak with candidates only outside of regular work hours.

It is also important to work with a "win-win" mindset and to be convinced that both the company and the candidate will be enhanced by their relationship.

A Typical Day

You can expect to keep long hours and to spend large amounts of time on the telephone either speaking with people or, more likely, playing phone tag with voicemail. As the assignment progresses, the search consultant will be traveling to meet with potential candidates. This is an example of a typical day for me:

- 6:00 A.M.: A conference call with the CEO of biosciences for a German pharmaceutical company to review top candidates for a market and sales position in the United States
- 8:00 A.M.: A series of phone interviews for a vice president of commercial operations in the Bay Area

- Noon to 1:30 P.M.: Lunch with a CEO of a bioscience company for a possible COO search

- 2:00 to 3:00 P.M.: Meet with CEO and board of a biotech company looking for a medical director (called "shoot out" meeting because I will be competing with other search firms for the business)

- 3:30 to 4:30 P.M.: Meet with individual who is frustrated looking for a senior management position and has never had to look; assist her with a career advancement program

- 4:30 to 5:30 P.M.: Member of BIOCOM committee meeting

- 6:00 P.M.: Return calls

DAILY FRUSTRATION LEVEL

As in any job, there are a multitude of things that can go wrong in a job search assignment. You may be working on five to eight search assignments that are at different levels of completion. Juggling those various activities can be a real challenge. I will highlight a few scenarios from my experience to better describe some of these frustrating experiences.

"You may be working on five to eight search assignments that are at different levels of completion. Juggling those various activities can be a real challenge."

Scenario One

After presenting three top candidates who match the position specifications perfectly, the top management of the company realizes that the position specifications need to be modified. This situation occurs because the management, during the course of the search assignment, does an in-depth assessment (often for the first time) of the existing skills, of projected growth and direction, and of the financial resources of the company.

When this occurs, the job specifications are modified, and there is generally a clearer vision of the needed skills for this position, but it often entails generating a new list of candidates.

Scenario Two

Your top candidate rejects the company's offer after you have negotiated for weeks and have come to an agreement. The reference checking usually is time-consuming, and coming to terms regarding the entire package takes creativity and effort. If the top candidate falls out at this stage, often you may have lost the second and third choices because of the time delay. It is likely that your top choice has developed cold feet at leaving a known environment and moving on to something new and different, but it is probably because he or she was offered a higher compensation package to stay at the current position. Often, you must start the search again.

Scenario Three

After extensive interviews with the top candidate, he or she backs out because the family decides that relocating from the east coast to the west coast will not work. Relocation is a major variable and always has to be discussed extensively since it is a lifestyle change. It is often a difficult process for the entire family to move, especially when they have school-age children.

Scenario Four

A candidate says that he or she is interested in the position you have described yet does not send the curriculum vitae (CV) as promised. If the CV is not forwarded, it is difficult to verify his or her interest and impossible to check background and experiences. Usually there is time urgency on a search assignment, and without the CV, you cannot include this person in your list of potential candidates.

Scenario Five

The candidate you brought into the company has had to take on more responsibilities and travel due to funding issues. The pace is too difficult, and the individual decides to move to another role. We have a 1-year guarantee for each search assignment, which means that if the individual does not stay in the job for at least a year, the search consultant must fulfill the responsibility and undergo another search at no charge to the client. This can happen regardless of how diligent and careful you are in the matchmaking process.

One of the most important elements of the search is to match personalities and corporate cultures. As a search consultant, you have the responsibility to assess the corporate culture and to bring in the key individuals who will fit into such an environment.

COMPENSATION, EXPERIENCE, AND ADVANCEMENT

Before I discuss a range of compensation information, it is important to discuss the difference between retained and contingency recruiting. Bente Hansen & Associates is a retained search firm, which means that the hiring company retains a search firm on a contractual basis to do the search, regardless of whether a hire is actually made. A contingent search firm gets paid on a per-hire basis. The fees to the search firm typically are related in some way to the annual salary of the position being filled at the client company.

Advancement with an executive search firm is tied to the amount of money that you bring into the firm and the extent to which you are perceived as a leader in your industry. Opportunities can range from positions such as the managing director of the firm's office or the managing director of a specific search industry, such as biotechnology or medical devices. Along with advancement come greater visibility and, hopefully, more search assignments.

The compensation in the retained search industry is generally related to the compensation package that accompanies the search assignment. It is financially more lucrative to search for a CEO versus a lab director.

At the top search firms, the usual fee that is paid by the client company is one-third of the estimated first year's total cash compensation of the individual who is hired. This fee is then divided into three installments: the initial retainer is paid at the start of the search, then the remaining two service charges are billed in 30 and 60 days, respectively. The final payment is often made when the successful candidate has been identified and has a signed contract.

As a smaller search firm by choice, we have had to separate ourselves from the larger group of firms to highlight our benefits. We only earn our second and third payments by achieving milestones, so the payments are not a guarantee.

The search consultant earns a percentage, usually between 30% and 50% of the amount that is paid by the client to the search firm. Of course, if you own your own firm, you keep 100%. Obviously, there are expenses you must absorb that are covered by a larger search firm. Most search consultants are paid on commission—they are paid when they make a placement—which means that the start-up period may be tedious, and the early earnings may be slim. With persistence, experience, relationship building, and successful search completions, you will build a client base that can equate to a solid six-figure income. Leaders in an industry earn in excess of half a million dollars.

Generally, the search consultant in a contingency-based practice has a market niche and has built up some loyal clients and followers who have been placed into decision-making roles. Advancement for the contingency practice is based on getting into an industry niche that is in demand and growing.

THE REWARDS OF BEING IN THE EXECUTIVE SEARCH BUSINESS

Before I entered into this industry, I did a personal skill assessment and thoroughly researched the field of executive search. Like many others, I have had the challenge of job hunting. I had some difficult and unpleasant experiences, and I vowed that when the opportunity presented itself, I would help people in this situation. Here is a list of instances that have helped others and me move forward in the industry.

1. **Helping others**
   I try to assist those looking for a job when I can. In most cases, the people I help are not candidates for the positions that I am filling for a client, so I can't offer a position. I usually can be helpful in revising a résumé to make it more marketable, targeting companies likely to value the candidate, offering contact names who may be of assistance, or suggesting a conference or workshop that would be beneficial in networking.

2. **Owning a business**
   Since I first wrote in the first edition of this book 8 years ago, I have learned a great deal and moved into a new phase of my search experience. Owning a company brings with it its own set of rewards and challenges, but it could be a natural progression if this is an interest.

3. **Receiving a monetary reward**
   Besides the monetary compensation, an executive search consultant must derive pleasure from serving as matchmaker between corporations and qualified candidates.

4. **Making a difference**
   Each person who is added to the management team makes a tremendous difference in the productivity of the corporation. This desire to bring together the right people with the right company for their mutual benefit is critical to being a successful and motivated headhunter. It is rewarding to see individuals find a position that matches their skills and their goals and allows them to be successful.

5. **Learning from meetings**
   Another reward is learning about a broad range of corporations and technologies. To sell the opportunity to potential candidates, you first

must yourself understand the corporate mission, products or science, and culture. You will spend a great deal of time on location at the client company, listening to and talking with persons who hold various positions in the company and gaining a real understanding of how that organization functions, its strengths and weaknesses.

6. **Meeting the key people in the industry**

A key reward is meeting and learning from senior people in biotechnology, such as Ginger Graham, CEO of Amylin; Tom Silberg, COO of Tercica; and Bo Saxberg, CEO of Strategic Services. They are leaders and mentors and truly care about the culture they are creating.

7. **Meeting with service providers**

This vocation provides you with the opportunity to meet and work with other service providers who often help each other in identifying new clients. Service providers, including attorneys, accountants, public relations groups and banks, are all needed by growing companies to help guide the management team and the board of directors.

In a rapidly changing business environment, search firms are taking on an expanding role in the companies they serve. As an extension of the company and a partner in search and to be highly valuable to the clients, you must keep up with trends and issues that not only affect that specific search but also add to your ability to influence succession planning, cultural fit, and leadership change in the company. I have had the good fortune to be able to identify strategic alliances that fit with specific companies and to help to fund start-up companies.

WHY THIS INDUSTRY?

Today the retained executive search business is a $10 billion industry because identifying and attracting the top talent is seen as the critical factor for growing businesses. The search industry allows you a career with a dynamic and growing environment and attracts people from all walks of life either hired right out of college or after professional experience. The outlook of this industry remains a function of the health of the economy and issues related to the FDA. In my experience, bioscience has been the strongest performing sector for the past few years, and there does not appear to be a significant change in the near future.

"With your knowledge of science, you are ahead of the pack in this technology-driven society."

With your knowledge of science, you are ahead of the pack in this technology-driven society. As you develop your career plan, build relationships early in your career and nurture them by keeping in touch with those you meet. You will have opportunities to do favors, and you will formulate your circle of business contacts. This takes time and effort, but the rewards will be great.

- A key question is "Are you a people person?" This career will take your knowledge of science into the less predictable world of people and leadership; you must have an interest in people interaction because you will spend a great deal of time on the phone.
- This industry also provides you with independence and probably is most attractive for people who like working as consultants as opposed to being a part of a large office.
- Financial rewards are certainly attainable.
- The position allows you to be deep within your specialization because that is a desire of the clients.
- You will find opportunities at a global level.

How to Enter This Industry

There are a number of ways by which you can enter this industry. A common way has been to gain experience in recruiting and in interviewing via the human resources profession. This is certainly one way to learn about screening candidates, conducting telephone and face-to-face interviews, and evaluating résumés—skills needed in this profession.

The other avenue is to work up through the management ranks and to gain experience with a number of different companies or job responsibilities. A necessary component of being a supervisor or a manager is to recruit and evaluate new staff. In this way, you can see firsthand the impact a new hire can have on a company. If you enjoy the research role previously mentioned, then this is a direct way to either take on a larger role within the research component or to move up to title of search consultant and, perhaps, partner. Another way to be introduced to the industry is to ask recruiters who happen to call on you. Be helpful and polite because you never know when you may be turning to them for an opportunity. I can guarantee that your name will be remembered if you have been helpful. Finally, there is a list of search/recruiting firms for your city available through Kennedy Information or through a business directory. Contact them directly or ask for an introduction. Most search firms focus on attracting leaders in their field, so industry experience is important to them.

Each firm has its own particular qualifications. Some look for industry experience; others look for relevant experience in managing and hiring key people. But the most valuable asset you bring to any company is your contact network. At an early stage of your career, build up those contacts—keep in touch, do favors, keep in touch, attend and speak at meetings, and keep in touch!

The size of the firm makes a difference just as in any profession. Small firms allow more mobility and an opportunity to do many things, whereas a larger firm may provide greater in-depth training.

PERSONAL COMMENTS

The search business is continually changing and evolving just as bioscience companies are maturing and starting up. I attribute the success I have experienced to my knowledge and relationships in the bioscience industry, my advanced degree in science, and my experience in a variety of management roles in biotechnology, medical device, and healthcare fields. The search industry is not one that is typically identified as a career alternative for people with science backgrounds. When identifying a future career or making a transition, it is wise to look at an industry with high growth, upward mobility, financial independence, and one that has a true appreciation for people's knowledge and education.

"The search business is continually changing and evolving just as bioscience companies are maturing and starting up."

Identifying the future leaders of our industry is not only a challenge but a contribution that makes a lasting impact.

19

· · · · · · · · · ·

CONSULTANT TO THE STARS:

Advising CEOs for Fun and Profit

· · · · · · · · · · · · · · · ·

Carol Hall, Ph.D.

Principal, BioVenture Consultants

Even though I had taken a classical academic science path—Ph.D. at Stanford in molecular biology, post-doctoral position at DNAX Research Institute in Palo Alto, California—my scientific career took a sharp turn away from the lab soon after completing my post-doc. I knew the time to leave the lab had come when I hated even the thought of pouring one more sequencing gel. The thrill was gone. Too many days in the cold room had left me permanently chilled toward the idea of countless more years of the same.

· ·

"I knew the time to leave the lab had come when I hated even the thought of pouring one more sequencing gel."

· ·

But what to do instead? I loved the intellectual aspects of science and was fascinated by the idea of creating new therapeutics to help patients. How could I promote that activity without having to personally run gels?

Keep in mind that what followed was not a well-planned career path but rather an evolving situation with random exposure to different pressures and opportunities acting as the Darwinian forces.

MY PATH INTO FINANCE

During my graduate studies, I took advantage of the close proximity of the Stanford Business School to attend a few courses, just to see what that world was all about. At that time, the late 1970s, the biotech industry was virtually nonexistent. This meant that most of the real job opportunities were in large pharmaceutical companies, a setting that didn't appeal to me particularly. While I didn't want to stay in academia, I enjoyed the informal environment that allowed easy collaboration and access to a broad range of disciplines.

I decided to do my post-doc at DNAX specifically because it was a small biotech company that would give me the chance to explore a move from the lab into the business side of a company. Unfortunately, I was there only a month before the company was acquired by Schering-Plough Corporation, and all the management was taken over by SP executives. It looked as though I was stuck back in the lab.

My big break came when my husband-to-be, another scientist, saw an ad in *Money Magazine* (*Science* isn't the only place to find interesting leads!) for a summer program offered by Wharton Business School at the University of Pennsylvania, to train people with Ph.D.s in the art of finding a job in the business sector. I took a leave of absence from my post-doc and headed for steamy Philadelphia.

Those 2 months were invaluable. I learned to speak a new language ("businessese") and how to pick up the phone and cold call for interviews. The course highlighted the first year of business school—an overview of economics, finance, marketing, and management. The finance component was the most interesting to me because it is very analytical and numbers oriented. A large part of the focus on finance was the role of Wall Street— this was the place to be if you wanted to be involved with raising money for the biopharmaceutical industry.

Unfortunately, these short programs, once offered by several leading business schools, aren't around anymore. A popular alternative is 2 years of business school, and I recommend that all aspiring consultants at least look at what these schools have to offer.

The most important skill that I acquired was how to pick up the phone and start looking for a job that wasn't listed in *Science*. After my crash business course, I quickly landed a job as a biotech industry analyst at a local San Francisco brokerage firm. During the next several years, as I moved from analyst to investment banker, I picked up many business skills that would later serve as part of the basis of our consulting business. These included the ability to analyze a scientific organization from the perspective of the business and investment opportunity it offered and the challenges this organization faced in raising enough money to realize that opportunity. I also gained insight into how Wall Street looks at science as opposed to how scientists look at it—very different views of the same world.

In addition, I took a 3-year self-study course to earn my chartered financial analyst designation. This C.F.A. substituted for an M.B.A. and gave me more creditability in the financial community. The C.F.A. is a credential that is well recognized among the buy-side and investment professionals—it means you have a minimum level of proficiency in certain key areas related to investment analysis. I loved being in the financial community. These jobs are fast-paced, you work independently, there is a lot of travel, and you are in a position to help a company achieve the next stage of growth and to reach its product development goals.

After riding out the aftermath of the 1987 stock market crash, I moved to a private leveraged buyout firm. These firms specialize in buying businesses with borrowed money in hopes of growing the business and realizing a big profit. After spending countless hours analyzing beauty parlor salons and meat packing plants, I realized that I had gone too far away from my first love—biotech.

BECOMING A CONSULTANT

The actual transaction to consultant occurred without much thought or planning. I had quit my job as leveraged buyout specialist because of a difficult pregnancy—that ride from our condo to the office was making me turn green on a daily basis. While talking to one of my many friends in the biotech industry, Cynthia Robbins-Roth, I learned that she had just landed a major consulting assignment in agricultural biotech, an area that I was familiar with from my investment banking experience. Over the past 3 years, we had spoken regularly about biotech financing issues, and I had written some articles on the topic for her newsletter, *BioVenture View*. This interaction made me feel comfortable that we could work together. We teamed up on an informal basis and completed the assignment in about 6 months. This first experience set the stage for our continued partnership, now in its sixteenth year.

Cindy and I are essentially freelancers; that is, we are self-employed and run a small business. This experience is very different from working for one of the large accounting firms such as Bain & Company or Andersen Consulting. All of my comments here refer to owning your own consulting business.

In our experience, most people who set up an independent consulting business end up taking a job at a client's company. Why? Because despite the rewards, there are many drawbacks to setting out on your own. Many people miss having an organization around them and the certainty of a regular paycheck. They dislike not knowing from month to month what projects they will be responsible for or whether there will be a project at all! Some people are very comfortable with using their technical expertise but don't like having to sell that expertise—the marketing side of the equation is important, or you won't have much work.

We have overcome many of these obstacles and you can too, if you know what to look for. If you decide to strike out on your own, the following sections provide examples of questions that will hit you early on.

What Are You Selling?

My partner and I both began working careers in the academic lab and in what were then early stage biotechnology companies. I moved into the financial community, providing services to the industry; Cindy moved from the lab into business development within a biotech firm.

In all, we built up roughly 15 years of experience and industry watching before trying to tell CEOs and venture capitalists how to run their businesses. Our biggest selling point is that we have grown up with the biotech industry, and we have been through several financing cycles. We have watched companies evolve from two-person start-ups to public companies with hundreds of employees, and we have worked with management teams as they grappled with the challenges of this growth.

This experience, and the strong personal contact network built up during that time, is useful to a broad range of clients: CEOs with "big pharma" (big pharmaceutical company) experience but no real exposure to entrepreneurial settings or working directly with scientists; academic scientists with no experience dealing with the financial community or business partners; potential investors hoping for insight to aid them in choosing the best opportunity to finance; big pharma looking for the best technology and team with whom to partner.

At BioVenture Consultants (BVC), we also are selling our scientific expertise, but more importantly we are selling our broad perspective of the drug development process, that is, how to take good science and turn it into a commercial product. As time goes by, our lab skills have become more and more antiquated, but our understanding of the scientific process is still very applicable. The ability to provide critical evaluation of potential new projects, to objectively review an R&D plan, and to help a client manage a scientific collaboration is a very important part of the services BVC provides.

We also have honed our writing skills, a dying art in this country, so we can turn out a good business plan quickly. Communication is key, whether with potential investors, potential key employees, or the business press.

Other areas where we have seen consultants flourish is in the clinical trial and regulatory area (backgrounds in the FDA or in clinical trial management), in public relations or investor relations (sometimes the two fields overlap), and in arranging partnerships between biotech and big pharma (consultants here usually have business development expertise).

Do You Take on a Partner?

Give serious thought to teaming up with someone. One of the biggest drawbacks to the consulting life is that it can get fairly lonely. If you are having trouble with a client, whom do you call? There is nothing better than a partner who can share your woes (and triumphs!). In addition to listening to you, a partner can cover for you when you go on vacation, and, more importantly, he or she can tell you if your ideas are sound. A day-long meeting is much easier to handle if there are two of you. Being "on" for 8 hours during a client meeting is tough work, and a partner is invaluable during these times. In addition, a partner with complementary experience and education can extend the areas in which your firm can operate with confidence.

But having a partner is work. Problems can arise when splitting up work (and fees) and handling the day-to-day affairs of the business. We have seen partners put together lengthy formally documented partnership arrangements, only to see them fall apart in a few years.

We have taken the informal route—there is no written document spelling out how we will work together. Each assignment is divided based on who has time available and the skills required. This approach has worked well because we had the luxury of time to work out our relationship, and we have a lot of confidence in each other's abilities and character.

The consulting partnership started as a part-time affair and was that way for the first couple of years, while our children were infants and Cindy got her publishing business more established. By the time BioVenture Consultants became a full-time occupation for both of us, in early 1991, we had collaborated on about a dozen assignments and figured out how to work well with each other. Because we both have strong personalities, and we take pride in our work, it was important to find a way to work together and take advantage of our different strengths to create something better than anything we could have accomplished on our own.

This "getting to know you" attitude has been carried over into our consulting business. With each new client, we write a contract that includes a small "getting to know you" piece of work, which we bid fairly inexpensively.

This gives the client direct experience with our working style and our capabilities. If the client is happy with that, we follow that initial project with much larger projects. This approach has worked extremely well for us. We are confident that clients will hire us for additional projects. This allows us to lose a little up front and to feel fairly confident that we will make it up on later parts of the job.

On a typical day, we will talk on the phone about three times, e-mail once or twice, and fax/e-mail one or two documents back and forth. We have tried at various times to keep each other's calendars, but in keeping with our informal arrangement, it has not really worked out. We discuss important dates, and we have learned to be flexible if one of us forgets to let the other one know what is going on. One of our greatest challenges was to learn to coordinate our activities so we could leverage our time.

We have toyed with the idea of adding someone to our partnership, but the right person has not come along. If you are just out of school, one way of breaking into the business may be to find a group that wants to add a junior person.

How Much Do You Charge?

The best way to find out what a consultant charges is to ask people who consult in the same field that you intend to enter. Don't assume that all consultants are your competition. Most of us specialize in aspects of the business that are different enough so that we gain more than we lose from staying in touch with each other. In fact, clients really appreciate it when you admit that a project falls outside your area of expertise and you recommend another consulting group.

In the biotech management field, daily consulting rates range from $1000 per day (usually for more inexperienced consultants) to $5000 per person, per day. Sometimes there are "success fees" on top of the project fee, typically when you help the company raise money or find a corporate partner. In some cases, you can get part of your fee in stock or stock options that can provide a chunk of cash if the company is successful.

The income earned by consultants is extremely variable, depending on how much work you bring in and the rate you charge. A consultant with around 10 years' relevant experience and a strong reputation should be able to earn more than $250,000 per year. Keep in mind that you most likely will not be working 8 hours a day, 7 days a week; your fees have to get you through the inevitable downtime.

It is a real temptation to underbid your work when you first start consulting because it takes time to learn how long certain assignments will take you, and you just can't believe that anyone would pay you that much to do something that seems so straightforward. Remember, you spend a lot of nonbillable time adding to your experience and information base by following the industry, taking care of your business (paying bills, invoicing clients, fixing the fax machine), attending technical and industry conferences, maintaining your network of contacts, and generating new business. Your clients must indirectly reimburse you for maintaining your business. In addition, issues that seem intuitively obvious to you, thanks to your years of direct experience, are not obvious to many clients. You must value your contribution if you want the client to value it.

You can bill on a "time spent" basis or give a fixed bid for a project based on your estimate of the time required to complete it. You can be compensated with a combination of cash and stock in the client's company (source of a potential upside if you do a great job and the stock value skyrockets!). We currently bid most jobs on a fixed-bid basis simply because clients are more comfortable knowing how big a financial commitment they are making. After all this time, we have a good idea how long a particular project will take. If you bill on an hourly basis, make sure to keep close tabs on your time. You will spend more time working than you realize, and clients will sometimes challenge your claimed hours—be sure you can account for the time you spend on a project.

There is a great deal of satisfaction gained when the check arrives in the mail. In a regular job, you can feel that you are paid regardless of how much or how little you work. In consulting, there is a direct correlation between the hours you put in and the reward. It is very gratifying to feel so in charge of your destiny. The downside, of course, is that the check needs to arrive sometime. Consultants moan about times of "feast and famine," and it is true. If you don't have funds to fall back on (retainer clients or a working spouse), only careful planning will get you through the dry times.

Getting It in Writing Versus a Handshake

Over the years, we have developed a client contract that we insist must be signed before we do any work. You would be surprised at how many eager clients blanche when they see the contract. Just seeing it in black and white makes them get serious. We have found that clients sign about 75% of the contracts that we submit without significant changes.

Early in our business, it was difficult to demand a contract from clients, but now, if a client resists, we know that they are not serious about working on a significant project with us. It can become tense at times in the negotiation stage, but better so before you have invested any time rather than later when you submit the bill. "No surprises" should be the rallying call for consultants when dealing with clients.

If you would like to see a typical contract, call us—we would be happy to share it with you. Key components include a description of the work to be done, a clear outline of the time frame and fees, boilerplate legalese to protect you from being sued by third parties for something related to the project (this can be a real liability issue when you work on projects related to financings or deals), and an explanation of limiting your liability to a maximum of your fee (otherwise, someone could wipe you out). The contract will not protect you in the event of gross negligence, breaking confidentiality, or illegal behavior.

A contract is also useful in dealing later with the IRS. It is important to define *in writing* your independence from your client so you can reap all the tax benefits (and Keough savings) of being a small business.

What About Travel?

Even for those who live in areas heavily populated by potential clients, travel is an important part of the consultant's job. We travel at least once a month, usually across the country, to visit current clients, to pitch business to a potential client, to attend a scientific conference related to a project, or to give a presentation at an industry conference. We have clients in Canada and all over the United States, and we travel to Japan and Europe once a year for conferences and to visit companies.

Establishing yourself as an industry expert by giving strong presentations is a great way to keep in touch with your network and to market your services—which essentially consists of using your brain. A great presentation on an area related to your services gives people a "free look" at your capabilities.

If you are traveling for a client, he or she covers all expenses. Make sure you keep good records, both for the client and for the IRS! Don't abuse your clients by flying first class (unless they agree ahead of time) or by charging nonessentials to their account.

IT'S ALL ABOUT REPUTATION

• •
"The only real asset of any consultant is his or her reputation."
• •

The only real asset of any consultant is his or her reputation. Most of our clients do not find us through direct marketing efforts (we don't advertise) but through recommendations by their personal contacts in the industry. We are reasonably well-known in the industry, in part because we are frequent invited speakers and moderators at industry conferences but more importantly because we have worked directly with many key players. It is absolutely crucial to maintain ethical behavior at all times, to do your best job for all clients—even the ones who drive you crazy—and to maintain strict confidentiality. You will be privy to many pieces of information that, if disclosed, could materially harm your client—and could break SEC laws and land you in jail for insider trading.

There will always be some folks who just don't like your style or your "bedside manner." Don't worry about that—as long as you are clear that your work is high quality. Stick with clients who are comfortable with your personal style, and learn as time goes by what behaviors you might want to change. The relationship between client and consultant is very close while the project is underway, and trust must flow in both directions.

While I took a circuitous route to becoming a consultant, none of my former jobs was a waste. My philosophy is "If you don't try it, how will you ever know that it isn't for you?" Working to earn a living lasts decades, so there is plenty of time to try different careers—especially while you are in your twenties or thirties. In the end, all my jobs have helped me directly or indirectly to build skills that eventually were put to use in BioVenture Consultants.

So you want to know how the meat packing plants were helpful? Several of our biotech clients have been interested in acquiring various businesses, and my experience with both leveraged buyouts and investment banking has allowed BioVenture to lead these discussions. The experience gained while conducting these financial analyses is relevant regardless of the specific business sector—numbers are numbers.

In closing, the best thing about biotech industry consulting is that we are essentially paid to learn about cool new science from some of the smartest people around. We get to work with a new cast of characters every month, and we are constantly learning new skills. Our network grows every day, and we work hard to keep that growth going. We have reasonable control over our workload and can take time to be with our families and to have other interests. Most importantly, at least for Cindy and myself, we don't have a boss telling us how to do our job. We are our own bosses. And science remains at the core of our business.

• •
"In closing, the best thing about biotech industry consulting is that we are essentially paid to learn about cool new science from some of the smartest people around."
• •

• •
"We are our own bosses. And science remains at the core of our business."
• •

20

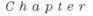

BIOMEDICAL CONSULTANT:

Specializing in Technology Assessment, Strategic Planning, and Grant Writing

Gail Schechter, Ph.D.
President and Founder, BioIntelligence

My career journey began in Bethesda, Maryland, where I grew up in the shadow of the National Institutes of Health (NIH). The NIH Clinical Center was the biggest red brick building in my world. This prestigious biomedical research institution captivated me from an early age when a relative was sent there for life-saving treatment. Combine the allure of NIH's edifice, my scientist father, and the thrill of my seventh grade prize-winning science fair project—a model of the brain with embedded lights for each major sensory area—and you can see how nature and nurture inevitably led me toward a profound interest in the brain.

Many moons have passed since that first science project. My path to consulting has been anything but straight. I worked for more than a decade at NIH conducting clinical research in biological psychiatry; was a speech writer for a high-level government official; administered a mental health clinical research center; was a clinical assistant professor at Stanford University School of Medicine in the Department of Psychiatry; worked at Genentech, Inc., setting up neuroscience collaborations; and finally, founded BioIntelligence, a consulting group specializing in technology assessment, strategic product planning, and grant writing.

For the most part, these transitions were smooth. Although my path was not preplanned, each job became a stepping-stone to something better. I learned that there are boundless opportunities to grow and flourish outside the ivory tower.

HOW I GOT THERE

I first attended graduate school in social psychology, which gave me a good introduction to the scientific method, research design, and statistical analysis. I became convinced that I was in the wrong field when we did an experiment to test the hypothesis that people throw down more trash on the street when the person in front of them throws down trash first. It was pretty tough to get excited about the outcome of that experiment. But what was I to do instead?

My whole career path shifted when an NIH scientist gave a seminar on studying brain function using electrophysiological brain recordings. I was excited to learn that there were quantitative techniques to directly study the brain. I latched on to the speaker when he finished his talk and asked if I could work for him at NIH. He said yes, and the next thing you know, I was working in the largest red brick building in the world!

As a research assistant in the Laboratory of Biological Psychiatry at NIH's National Institute of Mental Health, I was responsible for conducting clinical studies on psychiatric patients. I delved into brain function, transmission of electrical signals, effects of drugs on the brain, and relationships between brain structure and function. Our lab specialized in noninvasive brain imaging techniques, which rapidly shifted from electrophysiology to newer brain-scanning techniques, including magnetic resonance imaging (MRI) and positron emission tomography (PET) when they first appeared.

The NIH environment was characterized by a spirit of scientific inquiry, idealistic exuberance, cutting-edge science, relative scientific freedom, extensive collaboration, and access to the latest technologies. The downside included government bureaucracy, cramped working conditions, tense competition between and within labs, and budget fluctuations. However, I would enthusiastically recommend NIH and other federal biomedical agencies as an excellent learning opportunity and career step.

I am eternally grateful to my NIH boss and mentor, Monte S. Buchsbaum, M.D., who encouraged and supported me during the critical early period of my career. He introduced me to the joys of scientific experimentation and was a role model of an exceptional scientific communicator. Dr. Buchsbaum always told a compelling science story, and that skill has inspired me through-out my career.

After about a decade in the red brick building, I got kicked upstairs to the Parklawn Building and the offices of the NIH Extramural Research Program and the Food and Drug Administration (FDA). I became part of the staff working for the head of the Alcohol, Drug Abuse, and Mental Health Administration (ADAMHA), an umbrella organization encompassing three institutes. Gerald L. Klerman, M.D., fondly referred to as the "Chief Shrink of the Country," was a professor in the Department of Psychiatry, Harvard University School of Medicine, when he was appointed by the president to head ADAMHA.

Dr. Klerman also became a mentor extraordinaire. Thanks to my research background and organizational and writing skills, I became his ghostwriter. I drafted his speeches, coauthored book chapters, and pre-pared other documents. Each project required a great deal of background work, so I continued to hone my research skills. I learned and wrote about the history of biological psychiatry, intricacies of pharmacological treat-ments, benefits of psychotherapy, and design of large-scale clinical trials to evaluate the effectiveness of pharmacological therapy and psychother-apy alone and in combination. I got to attend high-level scientific meetings at the National Academy of Sciences' Institute of Medicine, where I was exposed to world leaders in mental health, to public health policy initia-tives, and to collaborations between and among government, academia, and industry. Once again, I benefitted from the opportunities available in the government, the rich learning environment, and a supportive supervisor.

A change in administration and the end of Dr. Klerman's tenure as a presidential appointee prompted my return to graduate school. I knew I wanted to focus on the hard sciences, but the most direct route was to build on my background and continue in psychology. I found the perfect graduate program at the University of California San Francisco Medical School (UCSF), where I could complete my psychology degree in one of the most outstanding medical schools in the country. To ease the transi-tion back to school, I obtained a leave of absence from my NIH govern-ment position and was awarded a public health service fellowship to pay my way.

Several years later, I emerged from this illustrious academic institution with knowledge of the basic neurosciences, including neuroanatomy and neuropharmacology, to add to my experimental psychology background. With my brand new Ph.D. in hand, I got a job at the Stanford/VA Mental Health Clinical Research Center, where I continued electrophysiological studies of brain–behavior relationships. This clinical research center focused on in-patients with major psychiatric disorders. This setting was an opportunity to gain valuable experience in conducting clinical trials to evaluate new drug treatments for psychiatric disorders.

Brain research continued its evolution from electrophysiology to the newer tools of noninvasive imaging, so when MRI came to Stanford, there was intense excitement. I volunteered to be one of the first to get scanned in a study comparing normal to schizophrenic brains. My MRI, pronounced "normal," is on my Web site in vivid color for all to see (www.BioIntelligence.com).

Because the Mental Health Clinical Research Center was funded by government grant money, I got my first introduction to both grant writing and reviewing. I was fortunate to find another great mentor, Ralph Peterson, M.D., director of the VA grant program. He encouraged me to participate in the grant review process, attend grant review meetings, and serve as a reviewer. I also want to acknowledge my Stanford/VA mentor, Walton T. Roth, M.D., a gifted researcher and hiker.

My academic affiliation with Stanford Medical School as a clinical assistant professor in the Department of Psychiatry and Behavioral Sciences enabled me to participate in the education of medical students, interns, and residents. My teaching duties included providing training in clinical research, teaching a course on brain imaging, and organizing journal review.

MOVE TO INDUSTRY

After 4 years at the Clinical Research Center, I was lured to my next opportunity. I happened to be in Washington, D.C., helping the VA with the grant review process, when an advertisement in *The Washington Post* beckoned me: "Neuroscientist to help with research activities for new Washington office of Italian pharmaceutical company." Although the ad said not to call, I immediately phoned the company and told them that I was the right person for the job, that I was only in town for a week, and that they should interview me immediately. Several interviews and one writing test later, and suddenly there I was, the new director of a neuroscience information network at Fidia Pharmaceuticals.

Was I really going to leave the security and longevity of my government tenure spanning two decades for this unknown quantity? I instantaneously decided yes, based on the opportunity to work for a dedicated neuroscience pharmaceutical company, try my hand at medical writing, and return to my roots in the Washington, D.C. area.

Fidia Pharmaceuticals, based near Venice, Italy, was opening a subsidiary in Washington. In addition to establishing a basic neuroscience center at Georgetown University, the company was opening a clinical research office. Ensconced in my first real office, decorated with mahogany furniture (after years of government gray metal desks) and an executive leather chair, I prepared monthly news bulletins, served as managing editor of a journal on neuroendocrine immunology, helped design clinical trial protocols, organized scientific symposia, published conference proceedings, and kept in contact with hundreds of international scientists.

When Fidia ran into problems with its clinical trials, I knew it was time to point my Italian shoes in a new direction. I spotted an advertisement in the back of *Science* for someone with neuroscience experience to set up research collaborations among a biotech firm, the NIH, academia, and other companies. After 23 interviews and a plane trip across the country, I was at Genentech working in the biotech industry in the early 1990s.

My job included evaluating novel technologies, identifying potential research collaborators, negotiating contracts, and arranging seminars. Genentech offered an academic-like environment, a community of stellar scientists, vast learning opportunities, and a successful model of drug development. Genentech had a unique culture that combined power science with a distinctive casualness. It was very intense and exciting to be on the inside, and anything could happen in a moment in the fast-paced environment. For me, the best things to come out of my Genentech experience were the amount of great neuroscience that I learned and the professional connections that still benefit me to this day.

As part of my work, I interacted with a number of small biotech companies seeking alliances with Genentech. One of those companies eventually asked me to consult on a strategic plan to develop a new approach to treating neurological disorders, which I thought would be exciting and a good experience. This consulting experience is how I went from working with the multithousand-person staff at Genentech to being a sole proprietor.

BECOMING A CONSULTANT OVERNIGHT

The request came suddenly one Monday morning from the CEO of a virtual company that I had tried to hook up with Genentech because of their complementary technologies to treat neurological diseases. "How would you like to consult for my new company," asked Gary Snable, founder and former CEO of Layton BioScience. The company was conducting preclinical studies, the preliminary data looked promising, and it was time start thinking about designing clinical trials to evaluate human neuronal cells to treat stroke. This company was poised for launch, and I was fortunate enough to be invited to go along for the ride. The thought of leaving the largest biotech company for one of the smallest was appealing. Everyone was doing it, so why not me?

My first assignment was to write a grant application to obtain funding from NIH to support the development of Layton's technology. We got the first grant and then at least a half dozen more totaling more than $4 million, and a new phase of my career was launched. Suddenly, I was a consultant specializing in grant writing. Even today, grant writing is the core of my business. From the time I wrote my first grant about 10 years ago until now, I have created a successful career in a specialized niche, been exposed to vast amounts of new science, and had tons of fun. I could never have predicted that this is what I would grow up to be.

A Typical Day

• •

"I start my day at the gym to exercise my body and my mind. I often get a whole new perspective and solve problems as a result of prancing about."

• •

I start my day at the gym early each morning to exercise my body and my mind. I often get a whole new perspective and solve problems as a result of prancing about. Back at my home office, I first attempt to tackle the toughest issues for current projects while avoiding telephone distractions luring me to new projects. Late in the afternoon, I do foray into new territory and eagerly listen to potential new clients as they chant their mantras. If it is a good match between consultant and client, then we do the dance of the contracts, eventually ending up with a signed agreement.

In addition to new clients, who typically hear about my services through word of mouth, I have several long-term clients who pay me a monthly retainer to do projects on an ongoing basis throughout the year. Most companies contact me based on referrals from pleased clients or colleagues. Networking at professional events is an important component of business development, and almost half of my business comes from this route. I do not advertise, but feel free to check out my Web site for further details (www.BioIntelligence.com).

BioIntelligence provides a range of consulting services. We specialize in technology assessment, strategic product planning, and grant writing. While grant writing is the core of my business, the other services come into play during the grant process. Each grant application takes from several weeks to several months to prepare, and a close collaboration between client and consultant develops.

Anatomy of a Grant

Most scientists are familiar with grant applications from our academic days when we would agonize over every detail and hopefully get funded. The majority of grants that I write are for small start-up companies desperate for funding of their research and development. In fact, NIH and other funding organizations have a special grant program that caters to small businesses (e.g., Small Business Innovation Research grant [SBIR]).

Let me digress briefly to extol the many benefits of grant funding for small biomedical companies. Grants provide an influx of much needed cash that can pay salaries, buy equipment, and hire consultants. This money is solely for the company, is not diluted, and requires no payback. Grants force a company to formulate a research plan, and that alone is helpful. Grants go through a rigorous peer review by experts in the field, so funding provides scientific validation and critical evaluation. Grant awards may also attract venture or other sources of funding in response to the scientific validation.

Writing grants has taught me many useful lessons in organizing and communicating information. First of all, a typical grant includes the following main sections: (i) specific aims to list objectives, milestones, and outcomes; (ii) background and significance to describe the scientific body of knowledge supporting the project; (iii) preliminary data to summarize results from previous studies; and (iv) experimental design and methods to provide the details of the experimental plan and analysis.

• •
"Writing grants has taught me many useful lessons in organizing and communicating information."
• •

From years of experience, here is a list of my top 10 tips to successful grant writing:

- Tell a story
- Engage the reviewer
- Anticipate questions
- Explain basic concepts
- Highlight the innovation
- Present the pros and cons
- Deliver the grant on a silver platter
- Go from molecules to new medicines
- Identify the pathway to commercialization
- Provide a clear, concise, compelling message

In my consulting practice, my approach to grant writing starts with meeting the company's scientists to learn about the technology that will drive the proposal. I read background materials provided by the company, as well as tracking down every bit of relevant information from the Internet, journals, conference abstracts, and patent filings. One important component is to assess competing technologies by evaluating what other companies are developing for similar indications. This information helps to highlight the advantages (and disadvantages) of the company's technology. The next step is to identify grant opportunities by searching the Web sites of the funding agencies to target the appropriate grant solicitations. There can be numerous new grant programs that, today for example, focus on biodefense for obvious reasons.

Then, it is time to start writing the grant proposal. In conformance with the recommended sections of the grant applications, I begin to formulate research goals, summarize preliminary data generated by the company, and develop experimental methods to evaluate the safety and efficacy of the new product. These activities typically take anywhere from several weeks to several months, depending on the complexity of the project. There has to be a close collaboration between the in-house team and outside consultants. There is a beneficial give and take that results in the best possible grant proposal. Typically, the company scientists are grateful for outside guidance, and we develop a close working relationship, and even friendship, from our joint efforts.

For preparing grant proposals, the time commitment varies depending on the proximity of the submission deadlines. The week before a grant deadline consists of total immersion to finishing a specific grant proposal on time, but the fortunate flip side is that other weeks are relatively free, allowing me to attend conferences, do volunteer work, or relax.

Grants are my mainstay, but I also do general consulting in product development, competitive intelligence, market research, and medical writing and editing ranging from company brochures to regulatory documents. A very enjoyable segment of my work involves writing overview reports on timely topics in neuroscience. These articles, prepared for industry publications such as *Drug & Market Development*, are a good impetus to stay informed on the latest research and provide tangible evidence of my scientific knowledge and writing abilities for potential clients. I get paid a flat fee to write these articles, but I am more than compensated by the opportunity to learn and to publish using my byline.

Taken together, all these consulting activities provide a grand opportunity to be close to science without being in the laboratory and to operate as a free agent with much flexibility.

The growth of my business, which has evolved over the years from one initial client to many clients across the country, occurred primarily by expanding my areas of expertise beyond neuroscience to include oncology, cell and gene therapy, drug discovery tools and, most recently, infectious diseases and vaccines. This expansion was made possible by partnering with scientists with specific expertise in these areas. I must take this opportunity to recognize my main business partner, Shauna Farr-Jones, Ph.D., a brilliant biochemist by training and the brightest, nicest, most sensible, most patient, and best teacher I have ever met. Her dazzlingly scientific explanations and reasoning are unsurpassed, and her ability to rise to new challenges is an inspiration. Shauna and I met at a networking luncheon at the San Francisco Bay Area Bioscience Center many years ago, and we have been working together ever since. I have acquired several additional partners over the years, and together we operate as a consortium of independent contractors, a business model that suits us all. We work as independent agents and also come together as needed to work on specific projects. In addition to scientific expertise and communication skills, I would say that the most important characteristics of business partners are dependability, perseverance, and a good mood.

I have considered several options for growing the business in new directions. It is a natural progression to expand my medical writing services to include clinical protocols, study reports, and other documents for regulatory submissions to the FDA. I recently have assembled an experienced team of medical writers to do more work along those lines. I found these experienced writers through networking and by contacting regulatory experts and asking for recommendations. Finding people who are trustworthy partners is essential. Payment can be a flat project fee or by the hour. Independent contractors are usually pleased when work is brought their way.

Another possibility for expansion is to reach across the pond to Europe by partnering with a colleague who heads a regulatory consulting company in Paris. We already have teamed up in the area of stem cell research and plan to collaborate more in the future.

What Does Consulting Pay?

Financial compensation for consulting varies widely, depending on the type of consulting (e.g., science analysis versus business analysis); how the information you obtain will be used (e.g., obtaining investment or research dollars for the client, creating a clinical protocol, moving a product closer to the market); and the experience, expertise, and reputation of the consultant. A good way to start is to talk about fees with folks doing similar consulting work in your area.

Consultants typically charge one of three ways: by the hour, by a flat rate for completing a specific project, or on a retainer basis—the client pays a monthly fee for a set number of hours per month. In the latter case, clients must "use it or lose it" because the monthly retainer is due regardless of whether they use the time, and they pay for any time over the allotted hours per month.

Early-stage companies often need outside help but lack the cash to cover expensive consultants. If you are a risk taker, alternatives to "cash only" fees include sweat equity—deferred payment based on future milestones or a combo of cash and stock in the client company. This can be tricky because you are putting your compensation under the control of others, and the future value of the stock rests in the hands of the company's management and investors. Be sure you have some level of confidence in the clients before agreeing to the cash/stock option. Of course, you are always taking some risk with this. But, often, it can be worth it to work with interesting people and exciting technology. No matter which fee option you choose, it must be comfortable for both you and your client to avoid bad feelings later on.

One of the biggest financial considerations associated with independent consulting is the lack of benefits. Benefits that are automatically available for employees within companies, including health insurance and retirement plans, must be self-paid by independent contractors. Don't forget to check with the IRS—you will be responsible for calculating and paying quarterly estimated taxes because there is no employer withholding income tax from each paycheck!

Of course, the second big financial challenge is the lack of a guarantee of steady client (and thus dollars) flow. Most consultants experience some version of "feast or famine," with incredibly busy times alternating with quiet (and nonpaying) down periods. Consultants are affected by economic factors far outside their control, including financing cycles for their clients, changes in government regulations, and events on the international scene.

PROS AND CONS OF THE JOB

Being a consultant has both rewards and challenges. The positive aspects are that the job continually exposes you to cutting-edge science and interaction with bright, enthusiastic people; provides vast learning opportunities; earns a respectable living; and is great fun. Being part of the process that results in the development of new treatments and improves patient health is a huge source of satisfaction.

• •
"Being part of the process that results in the development of new treatments and improves patient health is a huge source of satisfaction."
• •

Being your own boss can provide a glorious sense of freedom. When I am outside during the middle of the day, I keenly appreciate the flexibility that my job affords. I love to create my own schedule and be in control. Because my work products are tangible, I feel a sense of immense satisfaction when I complete a project.

On the other hand, there are killer deadlines, especially for submitting grant proposals, and intense pressure to complete projects while juggling input from client staff not under your control. Your work is often critiqued not only by clients, but also by the groups they are trying to influence—potential investors, corporate partners, and so forth. Panels of experts scrutinize every grant application, exposing any weakness.

> "Your work is often critiqued not only by clients, but also by the groups they are trying to influence..."

As a consultant, you must have self-discipline because there is nobody to stop you from procrastinating, no 6-month reviews to let you know what work habits need tweaking, and nobody controlling the quality of the final product other than yourself. In any consulting business, small and large, business development is crucial to keep that flow of clients coming. It is dangerous to become dependent on regular clients and ignore potential new business. Those regular clients can suffer unexpected disasters in their business (think Enron) and leave you without a paycheck until you build up new clientele. Just as diversity in a stock portfolio is important for risk-reduction, it is crucial in a client base.

SKILLS FOR SUCCESS

If your goal is to become an independent consultant, I recommend that you supplement your academic training with experience in the biopharmaceutical (or whatever is relevant) industry and spend some time with a consulting company. This will give you direct exposure to the drug development process, proposal writing, and other essential skills. A common saying in medical school is "learn one, do one, teach one"; ideally, you should learn first, do second, and consult third.

> "A common saying in medical school is 'learn one, do one, teach one'; ideally, you should learn first, do second, and consult third."

Specific skills relevant to consulting are not unique to this profession. These qualities are critically important, in fact, not only for careers in science but for success in other professions as well. Here is my top 10 list of essential attributes.

- Communication skills
- Leadership ability
- Problem solving

- Creative thinking
- Project management
- Interpersonal skills
- Positive attitude
- Professionalism
- Sense of humor
- Graciousness

Character traits that are counterproductive include pushiness, impatience, and rigidity. Forcing an issue prematurely does not work. If a company is not ready to begin a project, let it go and hopefully the client will reemerge at a later time ready to proceed. I have seen uncomfortable situations in which these attributes have resulted in failure of a working relationship and the project when success was within reach. A healthy respect for the natural evolution of projects and "going with the flow" will ultimately get you where you want to go.

To enhance and expand your specific knowledge and skills, a multitude of educational resources are available. At the same time that you are developing new skills, you will have the opportunity to network with interesting people and find out what types of jobs exist in the real world. For example, I completed courses at the Tuft's Center for the Study of Drug Development, the Georgetown University Center for Drug Development Science, and the Drug Information Association. While attending these courses, I met officials from the FDA, CEOs of companies that subsequently hired me to consult, and many scientists with interesting careers.

Attending regular conferences in (or out of) your area of expertise, such as the Society for Neuroscience, might be a good way to transition from one scientific career to another. These meetings are attended by industry folks and academics. There are also many excellent conferences oriented toward the business of science. For example, today I received announcements for conferences on nucleic acids, psychiatric drug discovery, and inflammatory processes (all sponsored by Strategic Research Institute). The Pharmaceutical Educational Research Institute (PERI) offers an extensive array of courses, as does the Regulatory Affairs Professional Society (RAPS). Continuing medical education (CME) courses presented by leading scientists, but sponsored by pharmaceutical companies, are held around the country to update physicians and provide CME credit, but most of these meetings are free and fairly open. Conference calendars are available on Web sites; for biomedical and biobusiness meetings, check www.biospace.com and www.bio.org.

In the San Francisco Bay area, both the University of California at Berkley and the University of California at Santa Cruz offer continuing education programs in biopharmaceutical studies covering drug development, clinical trials, and regulatory sciences. Several local organizations offer informative programs, including BioSF (www.BioSF.org), BioE2E (www.BioE2E.org), and the Women's Technology Cluster (www.WTC-SF.org).

By now, you probably have figured out that strong writing skills are the basis of many alternative careers in science. To hone your skills, join the national American Medical Writers Association (AMWA), which offers many courses, or local groups such as the Northern California Science Writers Association (www.NCSWA.org). Contribute an article for publication in the myriad of science magazines aimed at industry. Don't worry about getting paid for these articles—you will benefit immensely just from having your name out there.

To build general business skills, take advantage of the information and courses provided by the Small Business Administration (SBA), and attend local entrepreneur-oriented events. To focus specifically on the pharmaceutical and biotechnology business, attend events sponsored by the Biotechnology Industry Organization (www.bio.org), or wrangle an invitation to attend one of the major investment group's life sciences conferences, such as J.P. Morgan Chase H&Q.

Volunteering can be a useful avenue to gain valuable experience and expand your network. I am on the board of a local hospital and a supporter of many patient advocacy groups, including the Multiple Sclerosis Society, the Amyotrophic Lateral Sclerosis Association, and the National Stroke Association. Participation in such organizations can provide opportunities to learn about medical breakthroughs, connect with individuals with similar interests, find out about job openings and, most of all, feel good about helping others.

MENTORING

Mentors have been crucial to my career, and I am always trying to give back in some measure. The encouragement and patience of my early supervisors at NIH, who gave me a chance in spite of my flagrant naïveté and lack of experience, were essential to my career development. How are you ever going to get experience unless that first person gives you a chance?

Equally important to me was my mentors' ability to convey a sense of excitement about the work. It was a way of thinking and acting that encouraged me to live and breathe science. These same people served as role models, especially for communication skills, so that it was possible to learn just by watching them in action.

Following the lead of my esteemed mentors, I try to give back and to be helpful, especially to those scientists just starting out. As an added benefit, you can learn from those you mentor because they have more current training and are often smarter than you. Some of my mentoring efforts include speaking at UCSF Career Fair/Biotechnology Day on the topic of maximizing your career potential, presenting medical writing workshops at UCSF, participating in career mentoring programs at UCSF, conducting mock interviews with foreign doctors, and providing individual career coaching to the many scientists who call me for advice (Career@BioIntelligence.com).

Cori Gorman, Ph.D., a former Genentech scientist, created a fabulously valuable organization called the Women's Technology Cluster (www.WTC-SF.org). Gorman and WTC-SF have been catalysts for developing an incubator and providing support services to emerging companies. Whereas the group started as a way to directly benefit women entrepreneurs, the organization is now gender neutral. Cori and I have worked closely together on various projects to enhance the skills of start-up companies, including teaching grant-writing workshops to spread the gospel.

BLURRING THE BOUNDARIES

In contrast to the old days when academia was the only ivory tower in town and industry science was definitely considered second-class and a cop-out, times have changed dramatically. Today, there is a permeable membrane between academia, industry, and government, and nutrients flow effortlessly back and forth. A major change is the flourishing of post-doctoral positions in industry, giving young scientists exposure to the science of business and the business of science. With the availability of post-docs at NIH as well, there is a whole new generation of scientists finishing their education outside of the ivory tower.

Another indication of the importance of collaborations among government, academia, and industry was the federal government's response to the SARS outbreak. The government immediately called on leaders from industry and academia to mount a joint attack on the problem. The alphabet soup people (NIH, CDC, DOD, and FDA) also are pouring extensive resources into biodefense initiatives in an effort to find a recipe for national safety. This translates into increased government funding opportunities for industry and academia and a unique chance for major collaborative efforts.

The entire technology transfer field has become more sophisticated because the government and universities recognize the challenges of drug development and turn to industry to commercialize their inventions. In the field of technology transfer, there are major employment opportunities that build on bench science skills but offer a chance to leave the lab.

Many academic scientists sit on the scientific advisory boards of companies or create their own companies. Recently, several Nobel Prize-winning academic neuroscientists each started their own small company. Drs. Paul Greengard, Eric Kandel, and Arvid Carlsson, who shared the Nobel Prize in 2000 for their landmark contributions toward understanding basic brain function, are now entrepreneurs. Each has his own company: Greengard founded Intra-Cellular Therapies; Kandel founded Memory Pharmaceuticals; and Arvid Carlsson founded Carlsson Research. In addition, Nobel Prize winner Dr. Stanley Prusiner, honored for his discovery of prions, also started a company called InPro. Other noted examples in the neuroscience field include Dr. Floyd Bloom, an academic scientist who recently stepped down from his post as editor of *Science* and started his own company, Neurome. In addition, Dr. Zack Hall, noted academic scientist and former director of the National Institute of Neurological Disorders and Stroke (NINDS), started a company called EnVivo Pharmaceuticals and is currently interim president of the new California Stem Cell Institute.

WHEN ONE DOOR CLOSES, ANOTHER OPENS

As you can see from all of the stories in this book, once you have a solid scientific foundation, you can apply it to a wide variety of careers. As you build upon that foundation, every move is a step forward, and your accumulated experience defines you. As you gain more experience and wisdom (i.e., age), it is often where you have been and whom you know that is important. Thus, I encourage you to get the strongest possible education, set out in the direction that suits you the best, take calculated risks, and don't hesitate to change directions along the way. I am certain that you all will find satisfying and stimulating careers.

Having experienced the triad of government, academia, and industry, I highly recommend that you investigate the complete spectrum of potential science careers and perhaps even create one that is just right for you. I believe that being proactive and going after what you want is helpful, but I also think that being reactive and responding to job opportunities that exist in the real word is a useful strategy. It is important to recognize the role of serendipity—be open to unexpected alternatives and remember to look for the silver lining should your path get bumpy. Whatever career alternative you choose, it should feel good in both your head and heart and provide you with an opportunity to flourish in the garden outside the ivory tower.

I have the pleasure of ending on a joyous note. My client, with whom I worked to submit several grant applications over the past 9 months, just gave birth. She named her new baby "Grant."

SCIENCE CAREERS IN GOVERNMENT

21

· · · · · · · · · ·

SCIENCE AND PUBLIC POLICY:

Translating Between Two Worlds

· · · · · · · · · · · · · · · · ·

David Applegate, Ph.D.
Senior Science Advisor, U.S. Geological Survey
Former Director of Government Affairs, American Geological Institute

Science threads its way throughout the entire federal government. In any given session of Congress, there may be debates and legislation concerning air-quality standards, global climate change, and many other issues with a hefty scientific or technical component. In addition, Congress sets funding levels for the federal agencies that support or conduct scientific research. The range of issues addressed by the executive branch and by government at state and local levels is similarly dependent on science and technology. However, very few of the policymakers or policy-level staff in any of these settings have a background in science or engineering.

Historically, policymakers have sought the advice of the scientific community on issues large and small, and there is a long history of scientists providing expert opinion. But there is an equally long history of frustration and misunderstanding between policymakers who are looking for simple, straightforward answers and scientists steeped in uncertainty, multiple working hypotheses, and emphasis on detail. Policymakers are used to making decisions based on available information, whereas scientists loathe making a final conclusion, knowing there is always more data to collect and analyze.

THE NEED FOR SCIENCE IN POLITICS

This communication gap, combined with the growing importance of science and technology in society as a whole, has created a need for scientists who can work at the interface between science and public policy. What began (and still continues) as an advisory role done "on the side" of a traditional scientific career has evolved into a career in itself. A significant cadre of trained scientists now occupy the nebulous space between their colleagues in research and policymakers in Washington. Like scientists who pursue careers in the media, scientists in public policy are translators between two worlds, filling a critically important need.

The opportunities in science policy are diverse and are not easily defined. What constitutes a career in science and public policy (or put more simply, science policy)? A narrow definition would be those engaged in policy for science, essentially the management or administration of science itself. A broader definition includes all those working on science *in* policy, such as the input of scientific information into a wide range of policy issues and decisions that have a technical component.

Although understandably diverse, this group—call them science policy wonks—shares a number of qualities: they are good communicators, particularly as writers; they have an interest in issues outside their discipline; and they work well with a variety of people. The analytical skills developed through scientific training are equally useful in addressing policy issues. One congressional fellowship program for scientists listed desirable attributes for candidates as being not only a broad scientific background and strong interest in applying scientific knowledge toward societal problems but also a high tolerance for ambiguity!

Science policy is about advocacy, analysis, and advising. Scientists pursuing careers in science and public policy write speeches for members of Congress, develop environmental initiatives at the White House, manage federal agencies, and prepare long-term policy analyses at think tanks. They also advocate on behalf of their colleagues at scientific societies, provide issue briefs for advocacy groups, unravel regulatory requirements at consulting firms, provide technical expertise for law firms, and engage in a host of other tasks for other entities.

Because of recent budget cuts and the expectation of future ones, the scientific community is realizing that it needs to focus on Washington and work harder to justify its share of federal dollars. There is a growing recognition that an important niche exists for scientists interested in fostering communication between their community and the policymakers. Although professors still remain who see value only in cloning themselves, many more recognize that there is enlightened self-interest involved in putting scientists into policy positions.

MAKING THE SHIFT

"Unlike their counterparts in academic or industrial research, scientists in public policy often occupy jobs that are not exclusively reserved for their skills."

Unlike their counterparts in academic or industrial research, scientists in public policy often occupy jobs that are not exclusively reserved for their skills. Discussions over an academic faculty position might center on whether to hire a biological oceanographer or a physical oceanographer—a choice between a scientist and a lawyer is unknown. But many science policy positions can benefit from either of these backgrounds. Consequently, the scientist must make a convincing case for why his or her particular background is not only relevant but crucial to success in that position.

To use the analogy of a symphony, lawyers are the violins of public policy, since we are talking about formulating the nation's laws. Scientists and other technical specialists are the woodwinds, adding another dimension to the sound of the more numerous strings. Although few in number, scientists involved in policy provide depth and complexity to the sound. They are not and must not be considered the equivalent of Woody Allen's marching-band cellist in the movie *Take the Money and Run*. Far from being out of place, their expertise brings a critical and necessary element into the process.

In the past, science policy was something that a scientist came to late in a distinguished research career, either by virtue of getting "kicked upstairs" into administration or being asked to sit on advisory committees or other "blue-ribbon" panels that are still an important facet of the science policy landscape. These tasks were done as an aside and were not a career in and of themselves. Just like George Washington's ideal of a citizen-legislator, the scientists were expected to return to their laboratory after dispensing the necessary wisdom.

Today, those considering a career in science policy may do so at many stages, sometimes after only an initial training in science. For example, an undergraduate biology major who minored in government or interned for a home-state senator and subsequently lands a job on Capitol Hill is not uncommon. These people become part of the broad spectrum of professionals whose preparation includes a solid foundation in science, meaning they bring a scientific orientation and some knowledge of how science works with them to their job.

For a growing number of scientists, a career in science policy is undertaken following the many years of training and research leading to a doctorate. Some are drawn by a desire to see their training put to more immediate use and others by outside interests in political issues (such as environment laws, health care, or education). This chapter focuses on the post-doctoral route because it is the path I took and hence the one most familiar to me. But I also will attempt to address how to get started for both those at the undergraduate and graduate (or post-graduate) levels, as well as opportunities and challenges for a science policy career.

"For a growing number of scientists, a career in science policy is undertaken following the many years of training and research leading to a doctorate."

MY OWN PATH: TURNING A CONGRESSIONAL FELLOWSHIP INTO A CAREER

My route into science policy came through one of the few fixed points of entry: the Congressional Science and Engineering Fellowship Program. This program is essentially a 1-year post-doctoral appointment spent on Capitol Hill working with members of Congress or congressional committees as special assistants in legislative and policy areas requiring scientific and technical input.

Although administered by the American Association for the Advancement of Science (AAAS), the bulk of the congressional fellowships are funded by other scientific and engineering societies in a wide variety of disciplines. My fellowship was funded by the American Geophysical Union. Most require a doctorate or a master's degree with several years of subsequent experience in science or engineering. The sponsoring society is responsible for selecting the fellow and paying that person a stipend (which varies between $50,000 and $62,000). With their salary paid, the fellows come free-of-charge to work in the personal office of a senator or representative or for a committee.

This fellowship program was launched in 1973 in response to the lack of scientists on Capitol Hill and the perceived need for increased technical input in the legislative process. Between 25 and 30 fellows are chosen each year from a variety of disciplines. The program includes an intensive orientation on congressional and executive branch operations and a year-long seminar program on issues involving science and public policy.

The fellowships have launched many careers in science and public policy. Alumni of the program are well placed throughout Capitol Hill as staff directors, analysts, and professional staff members, as well as in high-level executive branch positions. After their fellowship year, about one-third of the fellows stay on the Hill or elsewhere in the Washington area in some policy-related activity. About one-third return to their academic or industrial origins, and the remaining one-third make some other kind of career change following their fellowship.

I applied for the fellowship while in the final stages of completing my doctoral work in geology, studying the tectonic processes that shaped the Death Valley region of California. My field area was about 30 miles from Yucca Mountain in Nevada, which the Department of Energy was studying as the likely site for the permanent disposal of the nation's high-level nuclear waste. I was intrigued by the technical aspects of the siting process—scientists trying to determine the potential for future earthquakes, volcanoes, or shifts in the water table that could create exposure pathways for the buried waste. My interest also was piqued by the difficult relationships among the scientists, the Department of Energy, and the many advocates for and against the site's suitability.

In addition, I have always been the sort of person who reads the paper every morning and tries to stay abreast of political issues. Having been a late convert to geology in college following several years as a history major, I still maintained a strong interest in the body politic, as well as planet Earth. The congressional fellowship was an opportunity to unite my diverse interests.

Plus, it was a job. When I obtained the fellowship, I was in a short-term post-doctoral appointment in my advisor's laboratory. Although I had a prospect for another post-doc out in California, it was not yet certain, and I had already experienced a number of rejected applications for faculty positions that went instead to those who had already put in several years as itinerant post-docs.

As a job, the fellowship could not have been better. Following an orientation into the ways of Congress and the federal agencies, I interviewed with a number of offices, meeting senators and representatives along the way. With my stipend paid for by the sponsoring society, the job market was considerably loosened!

I ended up with the Senate Committee on Energy and Natural Resources working on issues including Yucca Mountain, environmental cleanup of the nuclear weapons complex, the fate of science agencies in the Department of the Interior, dismantling the federal helium program (you probably didn't know we had one), and revision of mining law. With the partial exception of the Yucca Mountain issue, none were within my scientific expertise, but all required me to be able to process scientific information and then translate it in a usable form for the senators, as well as the committee staff.

As my fellowship year drew to a close, I decided that I wanted to stay in Washington and find a job in science policy. As luck would have it, an ideal job opened up, and my fellowship experience was critical to landing it. Following a brief stint as a regular staffer for the committee, mostly tying up loose ends, I became the rock lobbyist—an advocate for the geosciences with the more formal title of Director of Government Affairs at the American Geological Institute (AGI), a federation of geoscience societies. The job was a two-way street, seeking to inform and influence policymakers on issues affecting the geosciences and at the same time informing the scientists about policy issues in Washington that affect them. I never owned a single pair of Gucci tassel loafers, but I was a registered lobbyist, providing testimony before Congress and meeting with congressional staff and agency officials, both seeking and providing information.

A lot of time was spent writing—writing official letters, testimony, a monthly magazine column, electronic mail updates, and summaries of various issues. I was responsible for maintaining a Web site with information on environmental issues, natural hazards, resources, appropriations, and other policy issues that impact the geosciences.

After 4 years in the job, the editor of the Institute's geoscience news magazine, *Geotimes*, left. Because I was already writing a column and had run a newspaper in college, the executive director asked me to take over as acting editor, a position that quickly became a permanent second job. Like my policy job, being an editor required the ability to cover a broad waterfront of issues and get up to speed quickly on technical issues that needed to make sense to a nontechnical audience.

During the next 4 years, my policy efforts came to focus increasingly on natural hazards (such as earthquakes, floods, hurricanes), a policy area where the geosciences play an important role but one where political interest has a tendency to wax immediately after a disaster but then quickly wane once the cameras are gone. Along with my counterpart at the American Geophysical Union, AGI's largest member society, I formed a working group of organizations interested in supporting a congressional caucus with the goal of sustaining political interest.

The more I worked on natural hazards, the more I wanted to devote all my efforts there. And so a year ago, I leapt at the opportunity to take a newly created position at the U.S. Geological Survey as senior science advisor for earthquake and geologic hazards. I coordinate programs that run global and national monitoring networks; develop hazard assessments that are translated into building codes; and conduct research to better understand the processes behind earthquakes, landslides, and volcanoes.

When the Sumatra earthquake and tsunami disaster struck the day after Christmas in 2004, my first job was to explain the science of what had happened to the administration, Congress, and the media. The next step was to help formulate the policies that can be put in place to prevent such a disaster from occurring elsewhere.

GETTING STARTED: WHAT SKILLS DO YOU NEED AND WHERE DO YOU GET THEM?

Jobs in science policy require many of the same skills that make you a good scientist—research and analytical skills, the ability to handle multiple tasks, the ability to clearly communicate the results of your work, and a genuine interest in the subject matter. On top of that, you need the ability to work in a constantly changing environment. In most cases, you do not control the issues that come up.

A high premium is placed on the ability to write and speak well to a general audience and to work to meet a deadline. People skills are critical along with an ability to work with a diverse set of viewpoints. My job also requires management skills to maximize the productivity not only of myself but of those working with me. I still use many of the computer skills, if not the computer languages themselves, acquired through osmosis during graduate school.

Where do you acquire these skills? Many come directly from a person's scientific training; however, the ability to write clearly and persuasively about technical issues for a general audience is sadly not a common component of scientific training at the undergraduate or graduate level.

Other skills may be acquired from unexpected sources or avocations. Some of my most valuable experience came from working on and eventually running a newspaper in college. In contrast to the semester-long gestation periods for term papers or the even longer timescale for research projects, the experience of having to get a finished product out the door each week taught me about writing under pressure, editing and fact-checking, working as part of a group, and managing scarce time.

You can practice writing for a general audience in a school newspaper or write letters to the editor of the local paper. Meeting deadlines and working hard are also essential. One skill, however, can only be acquired once you have arrived in Washington: a high tolerance for acronyms (to match the high tolerance for ambiguity mentioned earlier). Maybe military training would help with that.

For the job applicant, it is important to realize that policy jobs are outside the research/academic sphere. A curriculum vitae is handy to have in reserve, but the résumé is the active tool for job-seeking. There are a number of excellent discussions about building résumés for nonacademic jobs, such as Peter Fiske's *Put Your Science to Work* (Fiske, 2001). As suggested previously, a person's nonscientific experiences may prove as useful as accomplishments in the lab, and the résumé should reflect expertise in computers, writing, and other skills with broad applicability.

Apart from specific skills and résumé techniques, scientists seeking a career in science policy must approach this new field with humility and the

• •

"Apart from specific skills and résumé techniques, scientists seeking a career in science policy must approach this new field with humility and the sense that they are there to learn as much as they are to teach."

• •

sense that they are there to learn as much as they are to teach. With all that you have to offer in technical expertise, the policymakers and lawyers with whom you will work can offer policy experience and political savvy. Some ways to develop skills and experience follow, and sources of additional information can be found at the end of this chapter.

Internships

For those at the bachelor's or master's level, there are many summer internship opportunities in Washington (both paid and unpaid) to work for Congress, federal agencies, nonprofit organizations, think tanks, interest groups, and other Washington entities. Congressional internships may not involve science-related issues but will provide an education in how Congress and politics in general work. A number of scientific societies, including AGI, offer summer and semester-long internships in science and public policy. Some of these internships are paid and can represent a summer job. Many colleges also grant course credits for internships. Closer to home, state and local governments also have intern opportunities. Internships are not lucrative, but they open doors and establish a track record.

Volunteering

Volunteering for a political campaign is another, very different way to establish a network of contacts—when they need a scientist, they will think of you. A fellow grad student at MIT became involved in Democratic politics in Massachusetts, worked for the Clinton/Gore campaign in 1992, and ended up as a senior appointee to the AmeriCorps national service program and several other posts. For those who do not feel comfortable with politics in its undiluted form, there are opportunities to volunteer with advocacy groups and science organizations that have more of an issue focus.

More School!

Because most science policy jobs require a master's degree or higher, acquiring the necessary skills may mean going back to school for an advanced degree in science or in science policy. For those already in an advanced degree program in science, consider adding a component to your thesis that addresses policy implications for your research. For example, a graduate student in hydrology looking at groundwater transport could add a chapter on the use of groundwater models in assessing contamination potential at Superfund sites.

A number of universities now have programs in science policy, particularly environmental policy. A master's degree in policy combined with a strong scientific background could make for a very effective and relatively unusual combination of skills. Many of these programs are geared toward working professionals, and it is possible to complete them while holding down a regular job. Although I do not want to advocate further proliferation of the legal profession, a science background combined with a law degree is another highly marketable combination in the policy world and elsewhere.

Whether in a policy program or in a straight science program, students with an interest in science policy should maintain a general awareness of what goes on in the world. When I was thinking about taking the Foreign Service Exam, the advice I received from a long-time diplomat was to read *The New York Times* every day for several years before taking the test, and I would do fine. Similar advice applies here. A general familiarity with the mechanics of government and the issues of the day will limit the amount of nontechnical information on which you will need to get up to speed and will minimize the likelihood of appearing to be a cello in a marching band.

Fellowships

The congressional fellowship programs are an important source of experience for scientists at a post-doctoral or mid-career level, but there are many more science policy fellowship programs sponsored by AAAS and other organizations. Like their congressional counterparts, these fellowships typically are directed at those with graduate degrees in science or engineering, they last for a year, and they provide scientists with the public policy experience necessary to obtain more permanent jobs. At the same time, they are an opportunity to make practical contributions to the more effective use of scientific and technical knowledge in the U.S. government and to demonstrate the value of science and technology in solving important societal problems.

Other AAAS-sponsored fellowships include the Diplomacy Fellowship Program in which fellows work in international affairs on scientific and technical subjects for a year, either at the U.S. State Department (10 fellowships) or U.S. Agency for International Development (10 fellowships). An Environmental Fellowship Program places scientists at the Environmental Protection Agency (10 fellowships). The Risk Policy Fellowship places scientists at the U.S. Food and Drug Administration and U.S. Department of Agriculture (5 fellowships) for a year as special research consultants, assessing the significance of environmental and/or human health problems through application of risk assessment.

Other fellowships include ones at the National Institutes of Health and National Science Foundation. One of the newer AAAS-sponsored programs places scientists in the Department of Defense (5 or more fellowships) for a year to work on issues related to defense policy, technology applications, defense systems analysis, and program oversight and management. Perhaps the newest fellowship places scientists with the Department of Homeland Security. Stipends for all these fellowships run from $62,000 to $81,000.

Some scientific societies, for example the American Physical Society, offer science policy fellowships that bring young scientists to work with the society's own government affairs program, again intended to provide the necessary policy expertise to complement the person's considerable scientific expertise.

A number of other fellowship opportunities are not specifically for scientists but may be open to them. Two similar programs on Capitol Hill are the Robert Wood Johnson fellowships for medical doctors and the American Political Science Association fellowships for (you guessed it!) political scientists. Scientists who are employed at federal agencies can participate in the LEGIS/Brookings Institution or the Georgetown University Government Affairs Institute fellowship programs, which places them in a congressional office for 6 months to 2 years.

The White House Fellowship is another program to consider. Started in the Johnson Administration, this fellowship recruits outstanding up-and-coming professionals from all disciplines to serve for a year as a special assistant to the president, the vice president, or one of the Cabinet secretaries. Among more than 500 alumni of the program, only a handful are scientists. Scientists have had a record of outstanding success in the program, but few apply, probably because it is poorly advertised in the scientific community.

The Presidential Management Fellows (PMF) Program is another outstanding opportunity for people right out of school. Every year, PMF takes from 200 to 400 people into a 2-year program that places them in Cabinet agencies, the White House, and Congress on rotational and developmental assignments. The goal of the program is to develop the government administrators and leaders of tomorrow.

At the end of the 2-year program, presidential management fellows automatically are converted to a permanent position in their agency, a unique aspect of the program. Scientists have been very poorly represented in this program as well, but the Office of Personnel Management and particularly the Department of Defense are eager for more applicants from science and engineering schools.

Most people apply right after a master's degree, through nomination by their school, but some come in after doctorates as well. The starting salary is on the low side, at a $65,000 to $69,000 level, but presidential management fellows are promoted to government service (GS)-11 after a year and then move into a GS-12 position after their internship.

POINTS OF ENTRY INTO A SCIENCE POLICY CAREER

Given the diversity of opportunities relating to science policy, there are consequently many trailheads that lead into science policy career pathways. Those at the earliest stage of their training as scientists have the greatest variety of paths to follow because they have more opportunities to adapt their education and are more flexible about salary requirements (i.e., will work for food).

For those who already are in the midst of their careers, an entirely different set of opportunities exists for developing the necessary skills and experience. You can become known among decision makers by demonstrating a willingness to communicate your expertise through your participation in National Research Council studies or on advisory boards for federal agencies. Certainly, the administration of science agencies is an opportunity for those who seek it, just as a deanship is an opportunity for those professors with an interest or flair for administration (or a knack for herding cats!).

This section reports on a number of possible pathways for people with a science background and experience gained through the internships, coursework, fellowships, and volunteering. All of these points of entry together represent only a handful of the many ways into science policy careers. The following paragraphs cover nongovernmental organizations (NGOs), Congress, and federal agencies in descending order of opportunities and experience levels required.

Washington is teeming with a motley assortment of nongovernmental organizations that occupy a somewhat nebulous zone between the public and private sector. Naturally, they are a haven for science policy wonks. Most of these organizations hold nonprofit status, although some may represent for-profit entities. NGOs tend to have fairly flat organizational structures. Although limiting the potential for advancement, these structures provide entry-level staff with a host of opportunities and responsibilities that more hierarchical structures (such as the Department of Energy, where it is possible to hold a job 20 layers beneath the Secretary!) do not allow. Several categories of NGOs have opportunities in science policy, including scientific societies, think tanks, interest groups, and the National Research Council.

Scientific Societies

Many scientific, engineering, and professional societies, as well as university consortia, are based in Washington, D.C. or have Washington-based government affairs programs. Many of the jobs are filled by individuals without a background in the scientific discipline they are representing.

The size of these programs varies from 1 to as many as 20 people. Scientists who apply for these jobs generally have some policy experience either in Congress or with a federal agency, part of the "revolving-door" world of Washington.

As with other types of science policy positions, these jobs are not reserved for scientists, and a scientist applying for such a position will be competing against other candidates who have considerable experience in government affairs as a career in itself, often having advocated for a variety of different issues and organizations.

I would argue that, ideally, scientists should be representing the scientific community. Otherwise, the advocate becomes another buffer between the scientists and policymakers. Having a background in the discipline that you are representing also provides insight into how issues concern or impact scientists and may improve other scientists' comfort level with the advocacy process.

Think Tanks

Another type of NGO is the so-called *think tank,* places like the Brookings Institution or Resources for the Future that provide policy analysis and advice to government and industry. Although these organizations tend to be dominated by social scientists, they address a range of technical issues that require a strong scientific background.

Although most of these organizations view themselves as nonpartisan, others (such as the Cato Institute) occupy a particular region of the political spectrum. A number of scientific societies also have policy-related programs that fall into this think tank category. Rather than advocacy, such programs focus on increasing the use (and usefulness) of scientific information in the policymaking process. An example is the Ecological Society of America's Sustainable Biosphere Initiative.

Interest Groups

Another well-known category of NGOs is interest or advocacy groups: think Sierra Club or National Rifle Association. Trade associations are a related group, often employing policy analysts and others to help make their case. Some groups such as Environmental Defense pride themselves on the number of scientists that work for them.

Although some of these jobs are in research, most are policy related or have a significant policy component. Working for a group with a clearly defined agenda may make some scientists uncomfortable, but for someone with a strong affinity for a given issue, working for an interest group can be very rewarding. For better or for worse, interest groups play a dominant role in informing and framing public policy debates and thus represent a tremendous opportunity for scientists who wish to improve the technical basis upon which these groups advance their positions.

National Research Council

The National Research Council is the principal operating arm of both the National Academy of Sciences and the National Academy of Engineering. Although it is congressionally chartered, the Research Council is not part of the federal government, but it does derive the bulk of its funding from Congress and from federal agencies. Much of the council's activity involves the preparation of reports by committees consisting of national academy members and other experts on a variety of science policy issues.

Although committee members are volunteers—one of the principal means by which scientists provide advice to the federal government—the council employs a considerable number of doctoral scientists to staff the committee studies and to develop new ones. These staff officers have backgrounds across the entire breadth of science and engineering disciplines. The staff plays a major role in shaping the reports and consequently in contributing to significant societal decisions.

The qualities that are most important in this post include a willingness to work in fields outside your scientific discipline, a love of learning about new fields, the ability to work well in teams, and, above all, being a good communicator who enjoys and excels at writing. The positions represent an opportunity to help define the agenda and to interact with all-star casts (hence, a certain deference may also be a useful skill). The Institute of

Medicine is the equivalent agency for the medical community with similar opportunities for those in health-related fields.

The staff officers are supported by staff assistant and associate positions that represent an excellent entry point for those with bachelor's or master's degrees. Those positions vary from heavily clerical to heavily research-focused work, so it is important to determine where on the spectrum a position lies when applying.

Congress and Congressional Agencies

Like NGOs, Congress has a very flat organizational structure. In a congressional office, even the interns are no more than three levels below the representative or senator for whom they are working. As a result, staff have a tremendous amount of responsibility and potential impact on public policy. Moreover, the turnover rate is high—the average tenure in any given job in a House personal office is under 2 years—so advancement can be rapid. The average personal office staffer is in his or her twenties and holds a bachelor's degree. Many worked on campaigns or interned before obtaining a staff position.

As an example, one of my first interns at AGI had just graduated from college with a geology degree. Based on her internship experience and an earlier internship on Capitol Hill, she obtained a job with her home-state senator as a legislative correspondent, answering constituent mail. Several months later, her boss became chairman of a committee, and she landed a job working on science education issues for the committee.

Committee staffers generally are older and experience lower turnover. They also are more likely to have a law degree or other advanced degree, but few have a technical background.

A number of scientists work for the House Science Committee, House Resources Committee, Senate Energy and Natural Resources Committee, Senate Labor and Human Resources Committee (science education and biomedical research), and Senate Commerce, Science, and Transportation Committee. Although many are former congressional fellows, others arrived from federal agencies or came to work in a personal office and moved up with time. In turn, many congressional staffers obtain policy-level jobs in federal agencies based on their Hill experience.

Opportunities also exist in two congressional agencies—the Congressional Research Service in the Library of Congress and the Government Accountability Office. The former is the principal source of information for Congress on every issue imaginable, including scientific issues and related policy areas such as the environment, natural resources, and health care. The latter is a watchdog agency, undertaking audits and other investigations into activities at federal agencies and elsewhere at the request of Congress. Although dominated by social scientists and assorted number-crunchers, the GAO addresses a wide range of issues that require a technical background.

Federal Agencies

In the United States, science is dispersed across many mission agencies with research conducted in support of program goals. That dispersal means that there is potentially a much broader set of opportunities for science policy wonks. In the European model, a single centralized science agency provides a single entity for research funding, giving scientists more influence in their own affairs but not beyond.

Although federal agencies are a natural home for science policy wonks, there are few points of entry. Instead, most scientists who have agency policy jobs either came up through the ranks from technical positions or came from jobs in Congress or NGOs. There is a variety of positions in science agencies and mission agencies in legislative affairs or as special assistants to high-level political appointees. Many of these policy-level jobs are themselves political appointments.

Although officially the hub of science policy in the federal government, the White House Office of Science and Technology Policy (OSTP) has relatively few opportunities for direct employment. Instead, scientists either arrive at OSTP with outside funding (such as a fellowship), on loan from their host agency, or as a political appointee. Scientists at OSTP are there either because they are experts on a specific hot issue or because they bring a broad background and understanding. In both cases, they have to be capable of writing speeches that contain good sound bites but keep the science accurate.

WHERE DOES A CAREER IN SCIENCE POLICY LEAD?

It may seem like an odd selling point for a career pathway, but a benefit of science policy is that it can lead all sorts of places, many of them not actually *in* science policy. As indicated earlier, many who do congressional fellowships take their experience back to their earlier jobs or go in entirely new directions.

Just as academic training is the coin of the realm for the newly minted scientist, so is policy experience, whether going back to academia, industry, or into a nonpolicy government research position. There are also opportunities in state governments at agencies handling environmental, health, resources, or technology issues. Having a firm understanding of the forces that are at play in obtaining grants, getting attention at the agency level or at the White House, and knowing how the political winds are changing are all invaluable to a business, government laboratory, or university department that relies on federal support.

For those who would like to return to academia (if not necessarily as researchers), it is possible to teach a course or two as an adjunct professor in one's scientific specialty or on science policy. There are also a growing number of programs in science policy, and it may be possible to secure a full-time position in the field, returning to academia in a different field from the one you were trained in.

For those who get the Washington, D.C. bug and want to stay in science policy, a number of the points of entry discussed previously can lead to long-term appointments. But these seldom lead to a lifetime job. As in most other fields, mobility and multiple careers are the norms for scientists who become science policy wonks. The high turnover rate in Congress provides opportunity but not necessarily continuity. Political appointments in particular have a way of vanishing in the wake of elections.

Although the flat structure of many NGOs may not be particularly conducive to upward mobility, opportunities do exist in management. Many of the same qualities that make for a good advocate are also valuable for leadership positions. Furthermore, experience in government affairs at a scientific society or interest group is readily portable and can lead to similar work for the private sector, federal agencies, or other organizations.

Law firms increasingly represent another potential avenue for scientists with policy experience. Just as Congress deals with highly technical issues in the process of making laws, the same holds true for those who interpret and argue over those laws. Many firms hire economists, engineers, and scientists to assist with the technical aspects of cases in areas such as environmental or intellectual property law.

Many of the opportunities that have been described focus on scientists providing advice and analysis to policymakers, but there is no reason that a science policy career should not lead scientists to become policymakers themselves. In contrast to the droves of lawyers and businesspeople in Congress, very few senators or representatives have a scientific background. Their small numbers include one geologist, two physicists, one chemist, and a couple of engineers, doctors, and veterinarians. One of the physicists, Rep. Rush Holt (D-NJ), is a former science fellow. Although numbers of scientists in Congress are few now, there are many races yet to run.

EARNING POTENTIAL

For the most part, science policy types labor firmly in the middle class with pay scales similar to those of their research counterparts in academia and government. That said, however, the earning potential can be significantly greater for those in the upper echelons of federal jobs, including senior executive service positions and political appointments, which can pay in the six figures. For those who leave the nonprofit or government sectors and work for government affairs offices in industry, compensation can likewise be considerable.

CONCLUSIONS

At a time when the emphasis among career planners is to prepare for not just one career but many, science policy is an important and fascinating choice to consider either as a diversion from one's present course or as an end in itself. Because it is broadly defined, many of the opportunities are there to be made. Science policy is a career field consisting of many niches, some of which are not readily apparent because the case for them must be made to other scientists and to policymakers alike. Although the lack of ready-cut positions and lines of advancement may seem daunting, any career field where you can make your own niche is one with a lot of growth potential and freedom to tailor a position.

Like one's education, policy experience is money in the career bank. The combination of scientific expertise and a firm understanding of how government works is valuable and marketable for jobs at consulting firms, large companies, universities, and within federal or state agencies.

Scientists are capable of much more than the specific laboratory techniques that they perfected in graduate school, and there is a very real need for scientists to apply their skills and knowledge to the public policymaking process. In doing so, they not only may find a satisfying alternative career for themselves but will help to ensure that traditional science careers for their peers do not vanish under budget pressures for lack of a compelling justification.

> "Scientists are capable of much more than the specific laboratory techniques that they perfected in graduate school, and there is a very real need for scientists to apply their skills and knowledge to the public policymaking process."

ADDITIONAL SOURCES OF INFORMATION

Online Information

- Additional information on fellowships is available from the American Association for the Advancement of Science (fellowships.aaas.org), the American Political Science Association (www.apsanet.org), and the

Robert Wood Johnson Foundation (www.rwjf.org). The Presidential Management Fellows Program can be found at www.pmf.opm.gov.

- Contact information for Members of Congress (www.house.gov *or* www.senate.gov) or the White House (www.whitehouse.gov) can be found on the Internet.

- Information on staff and internship opportunities can be found at the National Research Council and Institute of Medicine Web site (www.nas.edu).

- A good online listing of graduate programs, including science and public policy, is available from Peterson's (www.petersons.com).

- For one example of the type of policy analysis and advocacy done by government affairs programs, visit the American Geological Institute (www.agiweb.org).

- For more information on think tank activities, visit The Brookings Institution (www.brookings.org) or Resources for the Future (www.rff.org).

Hardcopy Resources

Fainberg, A. (Ed.). (1994). *From the Lab to the Hill: Essays Celebrating Twenty Years of Congressional Science and Engineering Fellows.* Washington, D.C.: American Association for the Advancement of Science.
Fiske, P. S. (2001). *Put Your Science to Work: The Take-Charge Career Guide for Scientists.* Washington, D.C.: American Geophysical Union.
Smith, B. L. R. (1992.) *The Advisors: Scientists in the Policy Process.* Washington, D.C.: The Brookings Institution.
Stine, J. K. (1994.) *Twenty Years of Science in the Public Interest: A History of the Congressional Science and Engineering Fellowship Program.* Washington, D.C.: American Association for the Advancement of Science.
Tobias, S., Chubin, D.E., and Aylesworth, K. (1995.) *Rethinking Science as a Career: Perceptions and Realities in the Physical Sciences.* Washington, D.C.: Research Corporation.

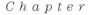
ECONOMIC DEVELOPMENT ADVISOR:

Building a Biotech Industry for an Entire Country

• • • • • • • • • • • • • • • •

Gina Lento, Ph.D.

Biotech Industry Development Advisor, New Zealand Trade and Enterprise

A JOB I COULD NOT HAVE PREDICTED

I work for the government of New Zealand as a biotech industry development advisor in its national economic development agency. With my colleagues, I run projects to create or augment the domestic infrastructure to help build and grow New Zealand biotechs and train Kiwi bioentrepreneurs, help them establish and fund their biotech businesses, and build the profile of New Zealand's biotechnology companies locally, domestically, and internationally.

Until Dr. Robbins-Roth asked me to contribute to this book, I had a hard time filling out that space on the airline departure card that says "occupation." I knew I had a cool and unusual job for a science geek, but didn't realize how much so until I began thinking how I'd describe it in a book chapter.

I never knew what I wanted to be when I grew up, and I can't honestly say I'm "grown up" yet, but I always knew science was going to be the means to an end for me. Like many science-trained people working in nontraditional but science-based jobs, mine was not a planned career path. In fact, I've had former employers ask me, "What *possible* value could that be to your professional development?" when I wanted to pursue some extracurricular activity. At times, I didn't know the exact answer to that question myself, but it's been sweet satisfaction to see how each of the things I did along my career path have prepared me for my present occupation.

How I Got Here

Originally from the United States, I got my first degree in biochemistry and cell biology with a minor in economics from the University of California at San Diego. During summers and part-time during school terms, I volunteered at a local hospital and worked at a small protein chemistry start-up company. There were only three employees at the company when I started. I ended up doing several things for the company besides the peptide synthesis for which I was hired, things like running the front office and building, selling, and installing the peptide cleavage machines the company sold. I graduated, spent several months backpacking around Europe, and then returned to San Diego to look for more work. This was back in 1988, shortly after San Diego started sprouting biotech start-ups like a rash. My experience at the peptide company got me a job at The Research Institute of Scripps Clinic, where I worked with clinical cardiologist, Professor Mark Yeager. Mark, with both an M.D. and a Ph.D., held a joint appointment in the institute's molecular biology department to explore the structure and function of the cardiac gap junction that he hypothesised played a role in the idiopathic myocarditis in some of his patients. Similar to the peptide company, our team in the lab was small. Just Mark and I were on the team, so I got exposed to a huge range of operational jobs and a lot of biochemical, biophysical, and clinical technology we used in our experiments.

The UC system had an education abroad program that allowed students to spend a quarter or a year at a university overseas to fulfill part of their degree curriculum. I wanted to do this but didn't have opportunity to during my bachelor's program. So after 3 years at Scripps, I applied for a Rotary International Ambassadorial Graduate Scholarship to begin another degree abroad. Based on some post-UCSD travel experiences of a friend who came to work with me at Scripps, I chose to take the scholarship in New Zealand. It was to be a 1-year post-graduate degree called a B.S. (honors), but it turned into a 12-year (and counting) career path.

At Scripps, while we were killing 40 to 80 rats every week to isolate and purify 1 mg of a very labile protein to study, the lab next door was doing some slick manual sequencing of portions of that same gap junction gene that was amplified using a new technique called polymerase chain reaction (PCR); they were hoping to develop a recombinant method for synthesizing the gap junction protein that I had been isolating from rats. They were using a couple of prototype models that looked like they came straight out of the Scripps machine shop. They were these giant water baths with interconnected plumbing to pump water at different temperatures to the rack holding the reaction tubes. The baths were attached to chart recorders showing the temperature inside a dummy tube. You *gotta* love cutting-edge biotech.

OFF TO NEW ZEALAND

So when I got to the lab at Victoria University of Wellington in New Zealand, I asked for any project using PCR in hopes of avoiding the ardour of vivisection. I was offered three and chose a project involving a genetic survey of the New Zealand sea lion and the New Zealand fur seal. Oddly enough, unlike the prototypes being used at Scripps, the New Zealand lab had two of the very latest new Perkin Elmer PCR machines, which we named Betty and Bob after a pair of crash test dummies we had seen on a car commercial.

The project was to identify genetic signatures for each different sea lion and fur seal breeding colony around the island. It turns out these endangered and endemic species are heavily impacted by normal trawl fishing operations, often decimating the population in any given year, and levels of incidental by-catch were suspected to be having a detrimental effect on population growth trends. The idea was to see if the provenance of the animals caught in trawl nets could be determined using colony-specific mtDNA polymorphisms. At the end of my B.Sc. (Honors) year, the New Zealand Department of Conservation was so impressed with what these new molecular techniques could tell them about the ecology of these animals that they offered me a fellowship to continue the work for a Ph.D. I finished a Ph.D. in molecular ecology and systematics of the pinnipeds (seals and sea lions) in 3 years.

Sometime during year 3 of living in New Zealand, I decided to become a naturalized citizen of the country, thus making me a dual citizen of the United States and New Zealand. I did it so that I could always come back to the country and stay as long as I wanted. Despite the fact I haven't left New Zealand yet, my dual citizenship has been very attractive to employers. Should they have need of an agent in the United States, they could send me there with no immigration issues whatsoever. My citizenship also affords me work opportunities in Australia with very minimal immigration issues, given the close relationship New Zealand has with Australia.

WHALES LEAD ME INTO A POST-DOC

At my thesis defense, one of my examiners, Dr. Scott Baker, offered me a post-doc at The University of Auckland to do a project in which I would use my molecular ecology skills for a different animal group, whales and dolphins. Dr. Baker had been approached by a nongovernmental organization (NGO) who suspected that the worldwide moratorium on commercial whaling that took effect in 1986 was, in fact, not working. The structure of the 1946 International Convention on the Regulation of Whaling actually provides a loophole allowing "scientific whaling" from which the "proceeds" can be sold. It was suspected that this legal avenue of whale meat sale was providing an umbrella for an extensive black market in the trade of whale and dolphin meat. The idea again was to determine the species origin (and geographic provenance, if possible) of samples of meat taken from fish markets, sushi bars, restaurants, gourmet department store, and even online mail-order houses, using mtDNA markers. The only problem was that the Convention on the International Trade of Endangered Species (CITES), originally set up to stop the illegal trade of elephant ivory, placed restrictions on the import of products from endangered species even for scientific purposes. But thanks to PCR and a CITES ruling in 1994 that synthetic DNA was not subject to the same import restrictions, Dr. Baker devised a way to amplify the native DNA from the sample in the country of origin and return the PCR product to New Zealand for sequencing and systematic analysis. Using technical advances in PCR machines, which were by this time based on Peltier-driven (read: really fast) heating blocks and engineered down to the size of a New York phone book, Dr. Baker put together the first portable PCR lab complete with electrophoresis boxes and a UV light table for photographing gels.

I joined the project in 1995 after Baker's first trips to Japan and Korea to carry on the "field surveys" of market samples of whale and dolphin meat. These were a series of very cloak-and-dagger missions held in very small Japanese businessmen's hotels; we used the method of coded knocks at the door to receive frozen chunks of meat in freezer bags from nervous locals. You can imagine how hard it was to explain to housekeeping why my bathroom trash can was dripping with blood and smelled of foul meat. Dr. Baker, who I will refer to from now on as Scott, had become friends with John Hansen at MJ Research (MJR), the company who made the small PCR machine, and persuaded him to develop a full, purpose-built PCR lab so we did not have to use our own suitcases and pack ethidium bromide-stained gel trays next to our toothbrushes. Soon was born the Mobile Molecular Lab

(MML), complete with a tiny centrifuge that looked like the Millenium Falcon. We, along with the Centers for Disease Control in Atlanta who were using the MML to test microbes in Antarctica, beta-tested the MML for MJR for 3 years through its early market releases.

Into Government Service

The results of our survey provided evidence for a black market in whale meat, and soon Scott and I were presenting to the International Whaling Commission's (IWC) scientific committee our research findings and the bioformatics database we had developed to track a sample from whale to dinner plate. I was asked by New Zealand's IWC commissioner (the former deputy prime minister of New Zealand, The Honorable Jim McLay) to serve on the New Zealand delegation to the main IWC political meetings as a DNA specialist while the members deliberated over the development of a forensic genetic tracking system to monitor illegal whaling. This was a fascinating experience. I spoke regularly with heads of state, government ministers, and other senior level government officials (even a prince) as we worked with like-minded antiwhaling nations to develop proposals and resolutions, as well as bartered on clauses and wording with the so-called prowhaling nations to get the resolutions passed. I watched masterful orators on the debating floor. I learned the rules of political engagement, such as counting the vote before the vote, and saw in living color the gripping, choreographed live chess match that is intergovernmental negotiation. The IWC went through a particularly intense period as the balance of voting power shifted from the antiwhaling to the prowhaling alliances, and through this time, it was serious edge-of-the-seat stuff. For those of you who have an interest in international law, politics, and environmental issues, there is no greater proving ground than the IWC. I'm sure there will be a movie about it in my lifetime.

I came to three important realizations during my time at the IWC that I have been able to apply usefully to other situations. First, the IWC debates are not about whales—they are about whaling. The lesson here is to make sure you understand perception from reality. Second, the IWC focuses on fishing regulations that the legislation put in place to govern an international resource (whales), which really serve as a regulatory precedent for all other commodities from the sea that can be traded. These commodities create much more valuable markets. The lesson here is to think of parameters, ramifications, and applications of technology (or legislation in the IWC case) far beyond the immediate arena. Third, the IWC doesn't only concern itself with science, it is also governed by politics. As naïve scientists, we thought all we had to do was show them the scientific evidence of illegal trade, and it would be a black-and-white decision to legislate against it. Hah! Were *we* young bunnies! The lesson here as translated to the biotech industry is that it doesn't matter how cool your science may be, there are commercial realities to deal with.

While it was a rare privilege to have my accumulated science to date appreciated in such an important practical way at the IWC (not always the case for academic research), I was becoming less enamored with having to write grants to survive. Getting invited to give papers and posters at conferences was nice, but it didn't seem like I was actually driven by those kudos. Finally, though I loved teaching in the lab and lecturing, having been the child of two school teachers, I saw that even tertiary educators are just as undervalued as primary and secondary teachers. More of the professional advances were tied to publications and grants than to the number of excellent students they produced. I began wordering if some commercial application of science might not be more fun.

I ENTER THE ENTREPRENEURIAL WORLD

My chance came soon enough when a colleague I had known for 6 years at The University of Auckland spun out his research into a biotech company. Professor Garth Cooper, discoverer of the hormone called amylin, cofounder of the San Diego-based Amylin Pharmaceuticals, and a Kiwi, came home to New Zealand in 1992 to pursue his research in the fields of diabetes and metabolic disorders. Though Garth and I had both been in the very young San Diego biotech industry in the late 1980s, we did not know each other there. But Garth knew Mark Yeager from Scripps, my first employer, through a long-standing collaboration with several faculty members at The University of Auckland. After some background checking with Mark and others, Garth offered me a position as VP of discovery in his new company, Protemix.

Again, it was a small operation; I was only the second employee and the first one to have an actual employment contract. Though I was employed to head up the discovery labs, there was so much work to do in the corporate office, and Garth recognized that I also had skills that could be applied to many of the tasks at hand there. I effectively, though unofficially, became the COO and took on jobs like developing employment contracts, intellectual property (IP) agreements, and Confidential Disclosure Agreements (CDAs) for all the university staff working for the company. There were several students undertaking research of commercial relevance to the company as part of their degree programs, but the university did not have a student IP plan, so I worked with the deputy vice chancellor's office to develop a plan that suited both the company and the university. I managed the full IP portfolio for the company and began developing an IP education program for the employees that would ensure proactive capture of all new IP. I convened the scientific advisory board meeting and even helped recruit my old boss, Mark Yeager, to the SAB. It was a nice example of life coming full circle.

The company was growing rapidly, and the product development of its lead candidate was swiftly approaching readiness for an approach to the FDA for clinical trials. The problem was how to establish a relationship with the FDA and find out to what division we should submit an IND. An old friend of mine from Scripps had turned her Ph.D. in molecular biology to patent law, and she started as a patent agent working in-house for Isis Pharmaceuticals. That was in 1990; she's still at Isis, and the company has now passed its 1500th patent application mark. I asked her to introduce me to the VP of regulatory affairs at Isis, which she did. I spent a couple of hours with him and learned how to find my way to the front door of the FDA and to navigate its Web site. There were several jaws to retrieve from the floor when I reported to the Protemix board that I'd cold-called the FDA and secured a decision from them regarding what division was most appropriate for us to apply to. This resulted in me being asked to shift to the development side of the company and begin writing INDs for the first two drug candidates. I also had the task of interviewing and recommending a U.S.-based FDA agent to shepherd the company through its applications to the FDA. The company also supported me through the first year of a postgraduate diploma in drug evaluation and pharmaceutical science. This coursework was an in-depth review of all my biochemistry and pharmacology, as well as a comprehensive overview of the regulatory process for getting drugs through clinical trials and approved for the market.

LURED BACK TO GOVERNMENT

As with all start-ups, there are financial rough patches, and Protemix hit its first one about 2 years later. I learned another valuable lesson: when it comes to "right-sizing," it is middle management that is the first to go. But one of the Protemix board members had met a new recruit, Peter Lennox, to the New Zealand government's 2-year old national economic development agency called New Zealand Trade & Enterprise (NZTE). Peter had been recognized as the driving force behind the exceptional achievements of a similar agency in Scotland—Scottish Enterprise—in building a biotech industry for Scotland. He'd been brought in in the great hope that he would do a repeat performance for New Zealand. A charismatic, Pied Piper of men (and women with his intoxicating Irish lilt), Peter had accepted the challenge to win the hearts and minds of New Zealand scientists, politicians, and businesspeople over to the belief that New Zealand could indeed play a role on the world stage of biotech. Anyone who truly knows the Kiwi mind-set also knows this is not as simple a task as it might appear. To assist Peter in this mission, a Protemix board member knew Peter was looking for clever, creative people with industry experience and specifically those who were *not* familiar with the civil servant *modus operandi* often found in large government organizations. Having seen my general outside-the-box approach to getting some of the Protemix operations underway, the board member recommended I go meet Peter.

I secured a coffee meeting with Peter, already notorious for being stretched for time. He asked what he could do for me. I said he could tell me his plan for introducing the New Zealand biotech industry to the world. He laid it out in 10 minutes and then asked again what he could do for me. I said he could give me a way to channel my passion for assisting Kiwi scientists to build biotech companies and play in the big sandbox with the global giants. Two things really gave rise to this passion. First, being American, I was inoculated with that unshakable confidence that anything is possible and had that way Americans have about them of waiving their own flag (which to non-Americans is considered obnoxious in the extreme). In contrast, Kiwis are incredibly humble and even quite reticent in certain situations.

Second, and integrally related, Kiwis are very clever people. In terms of patents and publications per capita, Kiwis are statistically the most entrepreneurial country in the world. But did you know that? If you did, it wasn't because a Kiwi told you. Or if they did, they didn't emphasize it in a way that got your attention. Through my peer tutoring at UCSD and my teaching during my post-doctoral position, I found I had inherited from my teacher parents a talent for convincing people of their own ability. I am a great cheerleader for supporting other people's endeavors. I felt if Kiwis were not going to shout their greatness from the hilltops, I would certainly be proud to do that for them. Peter had a sector specialist job available in his biotech team, a job that provided a very interesting vehicle for me to work with.

What Does an Economic Development Advisor Do?

I work with a group of people with similar backgrounds, in science (several of our group members have a masters or doctorate degree in some life science), in biotech (having spent many years working in the corporate offices of large and small biology-based companies), or both (like me, having started in academia and shifted into the private sector). We either work directly with biotech companies to assist them with aspects of business development or work on special projects to create the domestic infrastructure necessary to build and grow biotech companies. Such projects include things like establishing intergovernmental agreements with Australia to jointly promote Australasian biotech internationally and jointly fund Australia–New Zealand collaborative research in the private sector; writing a New Zealand IP manual; establishing a single national industry body; and developing educational, internship, and professional secondment programs. The range of things is quite large and stems from a series of recommendations made to the government by a biotech industry taskforce (www.industrytaskforces.govt.nz) that was convened in late 2003.

My particular projects are based around networking at regional, national, and international levels. I like to call it my "mandate to schmooze." I get paid to meet people, learn what they do, identify how they can add something to the business community, and hook them up with people who need their time and skills or recruit them into a larger work project designed to assist many busi-

•••••••••••••••••••••
"My particular projects are based around networking at regional, national, and international levels. I like to call it my 'mandate to schmooze.'"
•••••••••••••••••••••••

nesses. This latter aspect is referred to by many as "finding and fitting," sort of like playing Cupid. It requires enough understanding about people or companies to identify the appropriate person or company that can help them. For example, I have been the director for a regional industry network through its establishment phase. With its recent formalization and integration with the national industry body, the network will hire an executive director to take it forward, and I will move on to other projects. I work with my colleagues to increase interregional network communication through the newly established national industry body, NZBio (www.nzbio.org.nz) and its Web sites and newsletters, and by participating in the networking activities of one region and then sharing that information with other regions in New Zealand.

One special project of mine has been to develop and pilot a network of international biobusiness experts to assist New Zealand in building its biotech industry. It is called the World Class New Zealand network and is designed to build global competitiveness of New Zealand's biotech businesses through increased connectedness. Its members are hand-selected based on the relevance of their expertise to the industry and its specific growth needs and the member's ability to commit to active engagements on a philanthropic basis. The purpose of the network is to provide strategic advice to both the New Zealand biotech industry community and government, as well as to function as a virtual member of the NZTE Biotech Team. These experts contribute to the development of the New Zealand biotech industry by providing business advice, industry intelligence, development support, and entrepreneurial and educational support. They do this in a variety of ways: visits to New Zealand to meet companies; receiving New Zealand companies into their markets; working with New Zealand government groups; and doing onward introductions, professional consultation, as well as work with other network members on special projects. The work is really tailored to each person's expertise and available time. Through this network, I have been privileged to meet some incredible people, such as Ted Greene (founding CEO of Hybritech), Cindy Robbins-Roth (biogoddess), John Bedbrook (ex-pat Kiwi and CEO of Verdia), Juan Enriquez (Harvard Business School), Peter Andrews (Chief Scientist of Queensland), Brad Duft (litigated the first biotech case *Hybritech v.*

Monoclonal Antibodies, former general counsel for Amylin Pharm), and Murray Brennan (another ex-pat Kiwi and director of the Memorial Sloan Kettering Cancer Center).

Challenges

Winning the hearts and minds of people, convincing them to put sweat equity into a project, and convincing them of the value in participating in a program or networking event when they have the weight of running their businesses on their minds are many of the challenges. Convincing potential investors to learn about biotech is another one. In addition, I have to convince foreign investors to learn about New Zealand as a business destination, keep up with international trends in the industry, figure out how to market the defining capabilities of the New Zealand biotech, and keep up with the amount of reporting that government agencies require.

Rewards

Some of the rewards of this job include seeing a business succeed, finding funding, and signing a partnership agreement. I enjoy seeing success stories in the public media and popular press and having a government minister commit more resources to the biotech sector because he believes in the enabling power of biotech. I like watching a new contact's eyes light up when I say I'm from New Zealand. I meet new people constantly. (I collected more than 300 business cards in the first 18 months on the job.) The satisfaction when I introduce two people who end up doing business together, and they can't thank me enough, is rewarding as well. Having a prominent business leader say I've restored his or her faith in the ability of the government to help the company also keeps me going. I am proud when one of my professional recommendations is acted on; I also get excited when a new project that will somehow enable businesses to form or grow is conceived and when that project is bought into and resourced. I feel the sense of achievement when a project is accomplished.

WHERE TO FROM HERE?

Within the Agency

Technically, if an economic development agency does the job right, it does itself out of a job. If we create a vibrant, healthy biotech industry with a lot of financial backing and depth of infrastructure to accommodate a steady flow of jobs and significant value creation, we are creating the private sector environment for us to step back into.

I could not go up many levels higher and still do the kind of job I do, aside from a position called trade commissioner, which is effectively the same job but based in an in-market posting. The fact that I am a dual citizen does, however, make it very easy for me to expand my work for the agency into the United States.

The rest of the jobs at higher levels in the organizational chart are strategic, operational planning, and corporate and, in nature, have much of a human resources administration side; these are less hands-on when it comes to dealing with companies themselves. They sometimes focus more on high-level strategies to bring about legislation changes to align the New Zealand business environment with the relevant external markets. This can involve more interaction with other government agencies and ministers of parliament who hold key portfolios that impact the biotech sector than interaction with the companies. Government interactions are always more political, so if you do not have the patience and tack of a politician, higher administrative levels in a government agency are probably not for you.

That said, NZTE functions as the interface between biotech businesses and the government. As such, we have a mandate to think more laterally and move a bit more rapidly to address and assist the rapidly changing needs of business in our industry sector. Operationally, we have a fairly flat structure and work as closely with our director and general manager as with our sector specialist teammates.

Outside the Agency

In contrast to my previous job, where I was exposed to a thin slice of the industry through one start-up company's path from discovery to development, this job allows a rare insider's look at a large number of companies in all stages of development from start-up to well-established global traders. I am exposed to foreign and domestic CEOs; chairpeople; presidents; government ministers; heads of state; business experts; founding fathers and mothers of the industry; and the thought leaders of local, national, and international business networks. As such, it is the perfect place to learn about running private businesses. Depending on the amount of time spent in a sector specialist role, a person could return to one of many corporate executive level jobs in the private sector (e.g., CEO, COO, business development, IP management). I think anyone wanting to run a private business should do a training rotation in a relevant government post. Not only do you learn how the government views essential aspects of business law (e.g., corporate, tax, import/export, IP, regulatory) and funding (e.g., business development grants, academic and private sector research grants, venture investment), but you also get to meet and develop a relationship with the individuals running those programs, so you know who to talk to when you have a related issue in your business operations.

Other jobs that would be available to an ex-economic development advisor would be directors of company boards, independent business consultants, and industry association officers (e.g., the CEO of the trade union or local business round table). This is not to mention a whole slew of other government jobs, such as consul general to another country and staff member of an MP; depending on your educational training, this type of job on your *curriculum vitae* would make you very competitive as a corporate or IP lawyer, finance advisor, VC, university lecturer, or journalist, and the list goes on.

WHAT DOES IT TAKE TO DO THIS JOB: HAVE YOU KISSED THE BLARNEY STONE?

It takes a very extroverted person to be a biotech industry development advisor. You need to be able to ask questions of strangers and cold-call very important people and ask them to make a philanthropic donation of their time to a project. Or you have to convince people that it is in their best business interests to investigate a partnering or investment opportunity in New Zealand. Once you have hooked the suitor, then it is time to scrub up the bride. You have to prepare the client company to interact with this person. We are often asking the client to stretch beyond his or her comfort zones either personally or in terms of the growth of the business. Clients often need to learn something new, sometimes in a formal education setting, and it may have been decades since their last stint in a classroom. And not everyone is as dynamic a networker as they need to be. Then you need to create an appropriate setting for them to meet. This can be a private one-on-one meeting, a group instructive session, a monthly networking dinner (which requires the party-throwing skills of a socialite to keep it fresh, on topic, and attractive to people to attend and sponsors to pay for), a seminar series, or a formal university course. I have had done all of these things in this job.

So in general, you need to be proactive in engaging people in conversation and need to encourage them to interact with others. It helps tremendously if you're a good conversationalist. You need to have a fair amount of confidence in your skills and knowledge of the industry and courage of conviction to see things through when that initial spark of enthusiasm wanes. Networks, the ability to create and maintain them and link them into other networks, are critical to success in this job. I've been able to draw on relationships from every previous phase of my career path.

A Day in the Life...

In most government agencies, the legacy is to do your 9:00-to-5:00 shift and then turn off. The work ethic in this job is much different. My standard workday is anywhere from 8 to 16 hours, and when I am escorting important visitors on tour programs around New Zealand, it is 24/7 for the entire time they are in country. Fortunately, there are many times I can work from home, which helps balance the fatigue factor. You can have some fairly high-level meetings in your pajamas. The agency is organized around the "paperless" principle, meaning documents are shared across a database accessible from any site. We have offices across the length and breadth of New Zealand, and though I have primary responsibility for client companies in one area (Auckland), I can work fairly effectively from any office location. I travel domestically 3 to 7 days per month and internationally two to four times a year. I spend a lot of time on the phone and in meetings. I would estimate that 70% of my work is executed via e-mail. There are often meetings, teleconferences, or client functions to attend before or after hours or during weekends. The bottom line is delivery on projects and useful outcomes. I don't always have to be in the office, but I need to be accessible.

How Did Science Training Help?

• •
"A background in science is not an official prerequisite of this job, but I find it essential to deliver the best advice."
• •

A background in science is not an official prerequisite of this job, but I find it essential to deliver the best advice. You need to understand a company's technology and be able to explain it to a third party. If you don't know about the technology, you need to be able to read the company literature, figure it out, and ask the company's scientist to fill in the gaps. A broad knowledge of biotech is essential to map what general space a company is in and also identify potential areas of application for its technology. This, in turn, helps you match companies or individuals to others who may have complementary interests in the technology. But there are always areas of technology with which you're not familiar. In this case, the scientific training comes back as second nature: you jump online, go to the science or medical school library,

• •
"Most of the time, I still write scientist *in the occupation space on the departure card; it's almost like an ethnicity for me."*
• •

find an academic in the field, and just research it. Most of the time, I still write *scientist* in the occupation space on the airline departure card; it's almost like an ethnicity for me.

Our group is unusual in that five of us have a Ph.D. in a life science (in fields such as biochemistry, molecular biology, plant genetics, and environmental engineering) plus experience in health and biotech funding agencies, academic and government research or the industry, or both. Another two have a master's degree in a life science and experience in the industry. More often, economic development agencies are populated by business, economics, and political science majors. These people are a key ingredient of an effective advisory team as well, but in all my experiences on the job, the consensus of thought has been that it's easier to augment the scientist's background with business knowledge than to teach a non-scientist about biotech. So, as in many other jobs where science is not the traditional preparative background, having an advanced science degree is highly valued.

Both in hiring me for the job originally and in its continuation, the job has been molded around my specific qualifications. For example, in our strategic analysis, we have recognized that off-shoring is becoming increasingly important as the global industry uses it more and more in certain areas of drug development, especially in clinical trials. New Zealand companies and hospitals have some notable capability in drug development and clinical trials. In developing our operational plans based around these two facts, we have been able to create a key focus program to raise the profile of New Zealand's drug development and clinical trials capabilities with me as the program manager because of the drug evaluation degree I did.

So in recommending a course of educational or professional preparation for a job like mine, you don't have to be too prescriptive. I would say an advanced degree in a life science (for both the exposure to the technology and training in the scientific process of evaluation), some experience in the industry, and some notion of how government agencies work are the three main ingredients. Just as I've described about me and the rest of my team, a whole range of other experiences can contribute to what an individual brings to this job. As important as the background, however, is the right personality: this job requires a proactive, confident, creative, inspirational, or encouraging person with excellent conversation and networking skills.

• •

"This job requires a proactive, confident, creative, inspirational, or encouraging person with excellent conversation and networking skills."

• •

Chapter

23

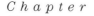

GOVERNMENT AGENCIES:

Directing Science in the Military

• • • • • • • • • • • • • • • • • •

Genevieve Haddad, Ph.D.

Director, Directorate of Chemistry and Life Sciences, Air Force Office of Scientific Research

My first job away from the bench was as the senior program manager for the Directorate of Chemistry and Life Sciences in the Air Force Office of Scientific Research. In that post, I managed a $5 million basic research in biology program for the U.S. Air Force, which focused on an area of neuroscience called chronobiology. This program supports basic research on the circadian timing system, the biology underlying fatigue, interactions of the circadian and homeostatic regulatory systems, and resulting individual differences and performance prediction. The Air Force supports such a program of research with hopes of coming up with information that can be used to develop new strategies to improve performance impaired by jet lag and shift work, night operations, and the loss of life and aircraft because of stress, inattention, or lack of vigilance.

My program included about 30 grants and contracts to top scientists at well-known universities, in industry, and in United States Air Force Research Laboratories. The scientific disciplines employed in this research included biochemistry, molecular biology, physiology, and neuroscience, as well as animal and human behavioral studies.

My primary duties and responsibilities included: (i) formulation of program needs and requirements; (ii) informing the relevant scientific community about the opportunities available in the program; (iii) encouraging submission of grant proposals; (iv) evaluation and prioritization of new research investment options; and (v) selection of projects for funding.

Part of this process involved peer review. This could include setting up panels or sending the proposals out to appropriate scientists for individual reviews. I determined which method of peer review and advice was most useful to me and then I implemented it. I oversaw all technical, fiscal, and administrative aspects of my program. I also was responsible for defending and explaining the program to management and to scientific review boards.

I was also expected to promote and coordinate optimal information exchange between the relevant scientific community and the operational Air Force, including training and education programs, technological development, and application of research findings. Not only was it important that I encouraged that these transitions take place, but I was also required to clearly document them as evidence of the usefulness of my program to the Air Force.

I regularly coordinated with my counterparts in other funding agencies to ensure a research program that met national policy objectives and avoids duplication. It was also important that I stayed up-to-date on relevant scientific and technical activities both nationally and internationally, including scientific progress directly within the areas we are funding at a certain point in time and also within related areas, and that I kept abreast of progress within my general area of expertise.

How I Got Here

I finished graduate school, taught for a couple of years, completed a post-doc, and then decided that I did not want to spend the next few years getting to know more and more about less and less. I liked the intellectual searching part of research, such as coming up with the research questions to ask, and I liked writing about results and interpreting them for publication. But I hated the actual hands-on experimentation, which I found boring and frustrating.

So what should I do? This was back in the days when every scientist around me, my thesis advisor, my post-doc mentor, and my friends all thought I was crazy at best, a traitor at worst, for wanting something different. After all, I was offered a couple of very respectable academic jobs; why would I want to do anything else? It must be because I was a woman and not really serious about science.

It was a pretty unpleasant experience, coming face-to-face with such strong prejudices. I was not able to find anyone within my academic world who was willing or able to help me explore other options. Somehow, through a long chain of personal inquiries, I was contracted by a United States Air Force officer at the Air Force Office of Scientific Research (AFOSR) who was looking for a temporary replacement for himself while he went off for a year at the Navy War College.

I didn't even know the Air Force funded basic research at the time. This was the early 1970s, and academia and the military were not the best of buddies. This officer managed a program of research in education and training, and he found out from the folks at the National Academy of Science that I might be interested in trying out such a position, that I was familiar with the scientific discipline critical to his program, and that I, in fact, knew several of the scientists funded through the program. I decided to try it for a year. Why not? It would at least give me a year of experience in grant administration.

So in 1979, I started an IPA (an agreement between a university and the government where the government pays your salary and the university agrees to hire you back after your stint with the government). The first day of work they put me on a military airplane and took me to Texas to listen to the three services defending their programs to AFOSR. I will never forget my reaction when I looked at all of those number charts and realized that the numbers were in millions of dollars. That first year, Jack, our boss, had already made many of the decisions about who to fund. However, he was very curious about my opinion of these scientists, and boy, did I have opinions. It was very different talking to brilliant senior scientists as their program manager than it had been from the position of a young, adoring scientist who had just received her Ph.D. But we were on the same side, after all, and I enjoyed every new thing I learned.

I put together my first program review of all these scientists, and I went to the annual meeting in my specialty as a very special person. AFOSR decided to offer me a permanent position. I had convinced my boss that the Air Force really needed a distinct program in visual psychophysics, which I was very capable of putting together and managing. And then I gave one of the best briefings of my life to the then-director of the organization, who said immediately after it that they should hire me fast.

And so began my career in the military. I enjoyed learning as much as I could about the Air Force and, for that matter, about the military as a whole. I started with no knowledge at all but had freedom and support to find out all I could absorb. When I decided that there was nothing I'd like better than

"I started with no knowledge at all but had freedom and support to find out all I could absorb."

to go to "war college," I received the support of the Command and was sent to the Industrial College of the Armed Forces (ICAF) for a year.

And what a year that was. The other students were U.S. Air Force, Navy, Army, and Marine officers, with a few civilians thrown in for variety. Never have I learned so much in such pleasant and stimulating surroundings. When we studied the Supreme Court, a few of the justices came in to tell us about it. Our studies of banking included visits with senior officers from the top banks in the United States. The general theme of the year was industrial mobilization for war and acquisition within the Department of Defense (DOD). These were the Reagan administration years, and the military was being built up. ICAF was a rare opportunity, one not to be missed if you ever get the chance.

After ICAF, I wanted a chance to use my new knowledge in something oriented more toward the Air Force than toward a basic research organization, so I took a staff management position at the headquarters of United States Air Force System Command as program manager in the Directorate of Life Sciences of the Air Force Office of Scientific Research. I became the headquarters representative for all applied research in the area of human systems. In this post, I planned, initiated, developed, and managed programs of basic research in education and training, human visual information processing, artificial intelligence/image understanding, and neuroscience. Each program included 20 to 30 contracts and grants to universities and industries. I formulated program needs, evaluated research proposals, and selected projects for funding; then, I oversaw all technical, fiscal, and administrative aspects of the research programs. I defended the programs though the 5-year budget cycle.

Gradually over the next 6 years, I was offered and accepted headquarters positions of increasing responsibility, always in some way related to research and development programs. I even spent a year on developmental assignment in the office of the Undersecretary of Defense for Acquisition. But staff work is not really my cup of tea, so when the chance came to return to AFOSR to manage a basic research program in chemistry and life sciences, I jumped, even though it was in an entirely different scientific area.

A Typical Day

There was no typical day—there were always new challenges. I had the freedom to structure my time pretty much as I pleased. Responsibilities shifted, depending upon the time of the year (some duties occur annually) and the needs of the moment. In addition, my responsibilities depended on my current interests. I interacted with a broad variety of people, from the most scientifically sophisticated Nobel Prize laureate to the youngest and most enthusiastic airplane mechanic. I dealt with the occasional politician; all levels of military war fighters; folks from the financial, contracting, and legal worlds; people from industry; movie directors; and toy makers. Some were very bright, and some were not. Some were flexible, and some were rigid.

All in all, I interacted with a much greater variety of people than I ever would have if I had stayed in a more traditional scientist's job. This was both exhilarating and a challenge. I couldn't expect most of the folks with whom I interacted to understand the experiences that shaped my thinking and decisions; their backgrounds and interests were very different from mine. I enjoyed this, but establishing a common ground for communication was not always easy.

I spent some days at the computer, sending e-mail to my principal investigators (PIs), answering e-mail requests about my program from prospective PIs, and designing briefings to explain and defend my program to those listed in the previous paragraph. Or I tried to sell a new program, answering numerous requests for information from a variety of Air Force management layers and oversight groups at the Office of the Secretary of Defense and sometimes handling requests from congressional staffers.

Other days I went to meetings. I attended from two to five scientific conferences a year, some very specific to the subject matter of my current program and some tangential and/or more general; some were even related to new areas about which I was curious and that I was considering adding to the focus of our program. Every year, I attended a variety of coordination meetings with my counterparts at other funding agencies to find out about their programs and to exchange ideas. Sometimes these meetings were actually turf battles. Of course, I also attended a number of nonscientific meetings. For example, one year, I was the organization's representative to a review board related to the reorganization of the Air Force laboratories.

Yes, managing a program of research for any of the military branches requires a large amount of travel—to scientific meetings, to university laboratories, to Air Force operational bases, and to Air Force research and development facilities. Many of the program managers here at AFOSR travel two or three times per month; some of this is discretionary, and some is required travel.

And most important, it was a requirement that I present my program at the meetings of a number of review boards—sometimes scientific, sometimes operational, and sometimes both. The purpose of these meetings could be to determine whether the Air Force would continue to fund research in this area or it may be to convince the DOD that the three military services have complementary rather than duplicative programs in an area.

I also organized my own meetings. Once a year or so, I had my grantees present their research to a review board I set up to evaluate the program on the basis of the science and for possible long-term Air Force application. Twice a year, I held a working group composed of scientists and Air Force operational types to exchange information. I wanted the scientists to develop an in-depth understanding of relevant Air Force issues, and I encouraged the operational folks to take advantage of advice to be gained from the brilliant minds of my researchers. Sometimes I put together a conference about a new area we were thinking of developing.

On some days, I read proposals and proposal reviews, made decisions about whom to fund, and then wrote the documentation necessary for our contracting people to write a grant. On other days, I read scientific journals and textbooks. I also spent the whole day on the telephone, putting out fires, keeping in touch, and making arrangements.

There are also other projects that arise because of current management interest in the topic. For example, one year our organization was very concerned with expenditure rates on grants. Expenditure is defined as the point at which the Defense Accounting and Finance System actually cuts the check in response to an invoice sent in by the grantee's institution. An understanding of this process was not originally part of my job before, but it became so. So I investigated. I tracked down how the process worked, where the kinks were, who had the relevant information, who could fix the problems, and how I could get to them. I'd hate to have to spend a whole lot of time on these financial details, but it was interesting to come to understand it and to solve the problems of concern to my management.

Several years ago, I was selected by the director of AFOSR to investigate and improve our agency's relationships, interactions, and image in all Air Force laboratories. The first year, I visited all the Air Force labs and made myself available for personal and/or small group discussions with as many of the scientists and managers as possible. I met a lot of people from a number of disciplines, and I listened and took notes. I learned a tremendous amount of science and application and about management and interpersonal issues. I wrote up and presented my findings and recommendations to senior management at all the labs and to management and all the PMs at AFOSR.

AFOSR implemented my recommendations, and our relationships with the labs have never been better. And I found myself with the additional duty of visiting these labs every year to make myself available to listen to problems.

Required Skills

To be a project manager of chemistry and life sciences, you need to be analytical, creative, and able to handle interpersonal interactions, to deal with computers and applications, and more. You bring what you are as well as who you are, just as you would to any job, and you use all of your talents and skills. What am I good at? Well, I think I am a very good listener. And I am pretty good at seeing the world from another person's point of view. This helps me figure out the best examples and the most appropriate kinds of arguments to convey my point. I am extremely curious about new things, and I like change and challenges. Repetition bores me, and when I am bored, I get mean. I am a pretty good briefer, especially if I have time to really prepare. I am able to take risks, make decisions, and live with the consequences.

"I am able to take risks, make decisions, and live with the consequences."

Training

The program manager job allows for on-the-job training. I was always training and learning new things, and I started more-or-less productive work my first day on the job. The Air Force is very generous about providing both part-time and full-time continuing education. I've been to war college, I have almost enough credits for an M.B.A., and I am able to attend scientific and management workshops and short courses pretty much as often as I like. Other program managers have taken sabbaticals to spend a year doing full-time research, to write books, and to become involved in diverse special projects.

Job Structure and Salary

Government salary structure is based primarily on the government service (GS) rating for a position. A top-level GS-15 senior program manager can make up to $116,517. Starting salary in government for a new program manager will depend somewhat on experience and academic discipline, but I think we occasionally hire at the GS-12 level, with a salary of $54,221 to $70,484 annually. Top salary for high-level managers, such as in senior executive service, is from $120,000 to $150,000, but they manage the managers of science.

There are many opportunities for advancement and for lateral job moves, but none are in program management. For example, I have since moved from program manager (PM) to director of the Directorate of Chemistry and Life Sciences. I have 10 PMs working for me, and they manage the programs, while I manage them. My current job description reads as follows:

Plan, direct, evaluate, and coordinate the $100-million United States Air Force basic research programs in the fields of chemistry and life sciences, encompassing such highly specialized areas as organic, inorganic, and theoretical chemistry and physiology; toxicology; biochemistry; molecular biology; neuroscience; biophysics; and human engineering funded by Air Force basic research funds and other money we spend from places like DARPA. Responsible for all operational, policy, and programmatic activities of the directorate, including all Air Force basic research in these areas and about 250 grants to AF laboratories, industry, and academia. Ensure that scientific merit is high and that goals are relevant to long-term Air Force needs. Encourage familiarity and promote appropriate integration of basic research into Air Force and other DOD applied research and development programs. First level supervisor/leader to directorate program managers, all highly respected senior-level scientists.

I have also held a number of other "lateral" government positions, some as training assignments and some because I actually changed jobs. These positions were primarily headquarters-type staff management positions that included developing policy and defending budgets and staff management of large programs of research. For example, in 1984 I transferred to the headquarters of United States Air Force Systems Command at Andrews Air Force Base in Maryland, where I spent 6 years in a variety of staff positions with increasing levels of responsibility and authority.

Headquarters staffers spend most of their time explaining and defending programs throughout the DOD and congressional budget cycles. I was responsible for a variety of basic and applied research and development programs, all vaguely related to the scientific disciplines I studied as a graduate student and a post-doc.

I also spent about a year in the Pentagon working in program integration and strategic planning for the Undersecretary of Defense for Acquisition. This was a fun job. The office was a small, very tightly knit group of people, including one Air Force officer, one Navy officer, one Army officer, one defense intelligence guy, one central intelligence guy, one civilian who came from the National Security Council, and me.

Half of us had scientific and technical backgrounds, and half of us had strong history and political science backgrounds. Our role was to integrate information about world events and develop both short- and long-range Department of Defense acquisition policy. We represented the Undersecretary in situations where national policy questions impact military acquisition programs in more than one specific technical area. For example, we integrated classified and open source inputs, and we wrote the technology sections of President George Bush, Sr.'s first major National Security Review. I also developed the congressionally mandated plan to use Department of Defense technological resources to help implement President Bush's national strategy to control the use of illegal drugs. It was great fun, and I learned so much.

WHERE CAN YOU GO FROM PROGRAM MANAGER?

There are a number of possibilities in industry, in academia, and in other government or quasi-government agencies. Large industries that deal with the government are often eager to hire an individual whose knowledge and contacts might help them. I am not referring to anything dishonest here. Companies are eager to have on board folks who know their way around the military acquisition of science and technology and of systems.

There are also opportunities in the so-called beltway bandits, or think tanks around Washington. Many of the military folks who retired from AFOSR have taken university positions, such as dean of research or provost.

A few have actually gone back to university teaching and research positions. There are always opportunities within other government agencies; I have seen advertisements from the General Accounting Office, the Office of Management and Budgeting, the Library of Congress, and even the Smithsonian Institute, for which I have exactly the experience requested. It would also be possible, and very interesting, to become a congressional committee staffer. There is a government program for young and eager employees of the executive branch to work "on the Hill" for a year or two.

WHAT OPPORTUNITIES EXIST IN THE MILITARY?

The United States Air Force is a large organization, and only a very small proportion of it is dedicated to science. The Air Force Office of Scientific Research is responsible for all of the basic research supported by the Air Force, whether at a university, within industry, or in a government laboratory.

At the moment, we have about 40 program managers. We seldom employ more than one scientist from a particular specialty area. Areas change from year to year and can be found on our Web site (www.afosr.af.mil). Areas in which we currently have research programs include those in the following list.

- Structural materials and mechanics of materials
- Particulate mechanics
- External aerodynamics and hypersonics
- Turbulence and internal flows
- Air-breathing combustion

- Space power and propulsion
- Metallic structural materials
- Ceramics and nonmetallic structural materials
- Organic matrix composites
- Electromagnetic devices, novel electronic components, optoelectronic information processing, quantum electronic solids, semiconductor metals, and electromagnetic materials
- Photonic physics, plasma physics, and imaging physics
- Chemical reactivity and synthesis, as well as polymer chemistry
- Surface science and molecular dynamics
- Chronology and neural adaptation, perception and cognition, and sensory systems
- Bioenvironmental science, as well as dynamics and control
- Physical mathematics and applied analysis, computational mathematics, optimization and discrete mathematics, signal processing, and probability and statistics
- Software and systems, as well as artificial intelligence
- Electromagnetics
- Meteorology and space sciences

SKILLS NEEDED TO SUCCEED AS PROGRAM MANAGER

Communication skills are absolutely essential for the effective program manager. I regularly explained and defended my program to higher level scientific management and scientific review boards and to a number of different nonscientific groups, in particular and most importantly to Air Force operational types, who have no time and just wanted to know the bottom line—what the research was good for and how it would help them. I also frequently had to explain program needs to the scientific communities involved, both in writing and verbally to individuals and to groups.

A wide range of personalities can do well in this setting. I'm an introvert, and I did this job well and enjoyed it very much. But I hardly think being an introvert is required. I suspect qualities such as independence, integrity, humor, patience, consistency, clarity of thought and communication, curiosity, and decisiveness are important. After thinking about this question for a while, I asked other program managers in my organization for their thoughts. The following is a sample of their responses.

- A strong interest and training in a scientific discipline

- A willingness to sacrifice the satisfaction of pursuing your own special research interests and ideas in that discipline

- The ability to tolerate and adapt to inconsistencies and frequent changes in administrative policies

- The analytical ability to understand the bottom line of complex scientific issues

- The ability to express the bottom line clearly in verbal or written format to others who may not have your technical training

- The ability to make decisions and execute actions based on those decisions

- The curiosity to explore and understand scientific issues outside your specific discipline

- The ability and inclination to interact with a broad range of scientists and administrators on issues of importance to them

• •

"In general, you must believe in your goals and take of position of strong advocacy to defend them."

• •

In general, you must believe in your goals and take a position of strong advocacy to defend them.

THE PROS AND CONS

I most liked being able to significantly influence the course of science—not simply through one discovery or one research project but, rather, by directing a whole program of research in the direction I believe is most profitable.

I least liked the many and continuous bureaucratic requirements that are repetitive and boring and that distracted me from my scientific program. The Department of Defense is a huge bureaucracy, and all of the niggling red tape common to any organization is certainly present here.

When coming to the military in the 1970s as I did, I never expected to find so many of the military officers to be highly intelligent, creative, well-read, cultured, sophisticated, and fun. Academics, at least when I was still in school, were convinced that the best and the brightest stayed in academia. I was pleasantly surprised and delighted to find that this is not the case.

But the two cultures are very different. At first, I did not enjoy having to dress for work—I wore jeans at the university, even when I taught. More seriously, academics are rewarded for questioning authority. In fact, a student has not really made it until he or she disproves the major finding of his mentor. Well, the military is not like that. Loyalty is probably the most valued quality in this environment. I thought I was showing that I cared by attacking all the weaknesses in the arguments of my government lab scientists. They were absolutely crushed, and they thought I was a terrible person who was about to destroy their projects. This is a real cultural adjustment, which I have only partly managed to achieve. I still question all authority.

I love "hair on fire" days, and I love stress; there still are not enough of those days for me. I do not like frustration, and any government bureaucracy has plenty of frustration. There are too many of those days.

There is a world of difference between academia and this position. In graduate school and as a post-doc, I did hands-on research—I made electrodes; stayed up all night with sick cats and sick computers; wrote proposals, journal articles, and scientific presentations on a very esoteric topic for a small, informed audience of scientists in the same or in a very similar esoteric field. My time was my own, dependent only on the requirements of the on-going study.

As program manager, I stayed up all night preparing briefings or participating in budget exercises. I also needed to respond to and be responsible for other people. The types of people with whom I had to interact were more diverse, and the communications process was a much more creative and exciting challenge. I had to translate my world into language that they understand, and I had to get them to care about my issues.

How to Get This Job

The best job listings for the military or government are found in *Science* and usually in the major journal of the scientific discipline being requested. *Commerce Business Daily* is also a good source. The key is to begin networking right now if you want to really learn what is out there.

The government is a maze, and it can be very difficult to navigate without insider help. I believe that most government jobs are advertised on the Web (www.fedworld.gov and www.USAjobs.opm.gov). There also are a number of fellowships available to get you in the door for a year or two so that you can learn about the structure and the culture of a position and decide if this is really for you.

The AAAS Defense Fellowship is a new option. In 1998, we awarded two of these fellowships, hiring a person for the Acquisition Office of the Secretary of Defense and hiring another person to assist the Deputy Assistant Secretary of the Air Force for Science, Technology, and Engineering.

The needed qualifications are a moving target. We seem to hire many more senior scientists now than we did when I was hired. I suspect that doing good science is the most important criterion. I would not have been able to do my job (nor would I have been hired) without having had excellent scientific training. Most important, my training and experience doing science taught me how to recognize good science. It also taught me how to talk to scientists, what to look for, how to start researching a new area, and how to understand whole science culture.

Because communication with a diverse population is crucial to performing the job well, it is critical to be articulate and to have the ability to explain science to the layman during the interview process. We do still hire IPAs (academic contracts) for 1-year assignments. And it is possible that it would help to become known as an Air Force laboratory bench scientist. There are 1-year government fellowships designed to give people a familiarity with government. One could also be trained in program management by taking a rotator position at the National Science Foundation.

· · · · · · · · · ·

APPENDIX:

Information Resources About Alternative Careers
for Scientists

· · · · · · · · · · · · · · · · ·

Cynthia Robbins-Roth, Ph.D.
Principal, BioVenture Consultants

In addition to the specific sources of information listed in the preceding chapters in this book, the Web sites listed in this appendix will give you many links to information about a wide range of alternative careers.

- www.geocities.com/CapeCanaveral/Hangar/4707/alt-careers.html

This site provides links to articles on science careers and sites with general information on career moves. You will also benefit from in-depth information about careers in law, tech transfer, public policy, writing and journalism, science education, and bioinformatics/biocomputing.

- www.sciencejobs.com

This is a Web site from *New Scientist* magazine, with a job database that includes a myriad of opportunities for scientists moving away from the lab bench; the site also includes jobs in academia, industry, and government.

- www.mbb.yale.edu/gp/gp_02d_ac.htm

This site is the Alternative Careers in Biosciences site provided by the Cellular and Molecular Biology Group at Yale. The site contains talks by former grad students and those with post-docs who now work in other fields. The Yale group also provides a wide array of links to useful sites, including the Young Scientists' Network, American Association for the Advancement of Science (AAAS) home page, Federation of American Scientists, the National Research Council's Science and Technology Policy Graduate Student and Post-doc Internship Program, the National Academy of Sciences Career Planning Center, the National Science Foundation, and the Tech Transfer Fellowship Program at the National Cancer Institute.

- http://nextwave.sciencemag.org/features/alternative_careers.dtl

Browse through this Web site that publishes the Directory of Alternative Careers for Scientists of *Science Magazine's* NextWave.

- http://gradschool.about.com/cs/alternativecareer/

Visit this site to view a collection of relevant articles, including *Alternative careers for scientists, traitors or trailblazers?*, *Deprogramming from the academic cult*, and *Where to find information on nonacademic careers.*

- www.biotechinsider.com/

This site works in conjunction with Medzilla, a job site specializing in biotech, pharmaceutical, healthcare, and life sciences jobs. You will find links to a wide selection of books to help you explore job hunting tools, recruiters, jobs in many aspects of these industries, and links to fun stuff like "The Dilbert Principal: Cubicle's Eye View of Bosses, Meeting, Management Fads, & Other Workplace Afflictions." There's also a salary database to query.

- www.elevateyourcareer.com/

You could benefit from the home of "elevations," a career assessment tool that looks at your values, skills, career interests, and personality and helps point you at career paths that fit with your unique combination. You can take the test online and receive a list of career alternatives that include job titles and descriptions of typical responsibilities. You are directed to Web sites where you can research those careers. This site also includes a career center, as well as information on workshops and coaching services.

INDEX

A

Academia
  lab v., 3–4
  leaving comfort zone of, 149–150
  transition from leaving, 150–151
Accounting, 73
Acorda Therapeutics, 97
Administration. *See also* Policy
    administration
  challenges in, 120
  as high-wattage activity, 120
Advanced Tissue Sciences, Inc., 97
Advertising, in publishing, 44
Air Force, research for, 279
Attention span, short, 18

B

Base salary, 166
Bates College, 3
Bayh-Dole Act, 183
Benefits, 236
BioAbility, 53
  growth of, 56
biochemists, protein, 3
Biological sciences
  biotech industry and, 2
  industry opportunities for people
    in, 48
Biomedical consulting, 227
BioPeople Magazine, 1
  creation of, 9

Biotechnology analysts
  attributes of, 90
  becoming, 91–92
  client relationships with, 87
  consulting done by, 83
  corporate financing as part of, 88
  evolving into investment banking, 65–66
  as fast paced, 84
  industry trends and, 87
  for investment banks, 63–65
  investment decisions by, 85–86
  job description of, 84–88
  job seeking as, 91
  limited jobs for, 91
  marketing stocks to buyers by, 86–87
  marketing trips for, 76
  M.B.A. for, 82–83
  networking for, 84–85
  positives/negatives of being, 89–90
  research by, 84
  salary for, 89–90
  scientific background for, 92
  on sell-side, 92–93
  skill set necessary for, 75, 92
  successful, 65
  typical day as, 76–77
  writing's importance for, 90
Biotechnology centers, 49
Biotechnology industry
  biological sciences and, 2
  business of, 8, 81–83